GORILLA FOOD

Living and Eating Organic, Vegan, and Raw

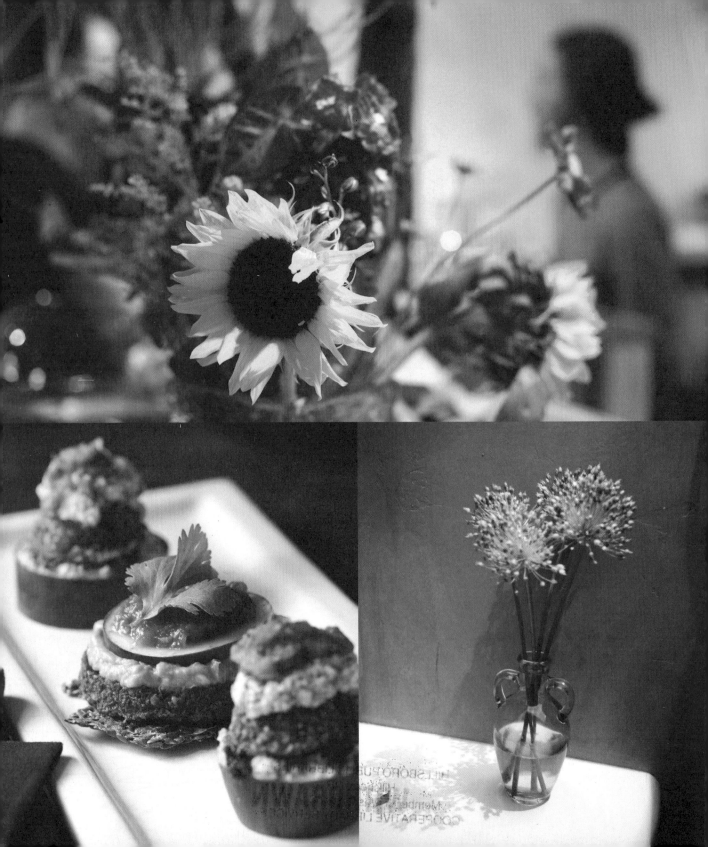

GORILLAFOOD

Living and Eating Organic, Vegan, and Raw

AARON ASH

ARSENAL
PULP PRESS

VANCOUVER

GORILLA FOOD
Copyright © 2012 by Aaron Ash

SECOND PRINTING: 2013

ARSENAL PULP PRESS
Suite 101 – 211 East Georgia St.
Vancouver, BC V6A 1Z6
Canada
arsenalpulp.com

The publisher gratefully acknowledges the support of the Government of Canada (through the Canada Book Fund) and the Government of British Columbia (through the Book Publishing Tax Credit Program) for its publishing activities.

The author and publisher assert that the information contained in this book is true and complete to the best of their knowledge. All recommendations are made without the guarantee on the part of the author and publisher. The author and publisher disclaim any liability in connection with the use of this information. For more information, contact the publisher.

Note for our UK readers: measurements for non-liquids are for volume, not weight.

Design by Li Eng-Lodge, Electra Design Group
Cover and interior food photographs by Tracie Kusiewicz, Foodie Photography
Restaurant photographs by Kyla Brown
Back cover photograph of author by Amanda Bullick, Brutally Beautiful
Editing by Susan Safyan
Copyediting by Angela Caravan

Printed and bound in Korea

5245 8528 9/13

Library and Archives Canada Cataloguing in Publication:

Ash, Aaron
      Gorilla food : living and eating organic, vegan, and
raw / Aaron Ash.

 Includes index.
ISBN 978-1-55152-470-2

    1. Raw foods. 2. Raw food diet—Recipes.
3. Vegan cooking. 4. Cookbooks— I. Title.

TX837.A79 2012   641.5'636   C2012-903262-X

Contents

I bow to all those who have reminded me to find joy in the service of humanity and to those who have reminded me that service is a path to liberation.

I feel blessed to be serving this food.

Acknowledgments

I am honored to share these recipes, many of which are favorites from the Gorilla Food menu. They stem from a love for being vegan and a joy for sharing food with others. They come through friendship, travel, synchronicity, and magic.

I give a lifetime of thanks for all of the amazing and inspiring people who have been a part of and remain Gorilla Food family.

I hope you will enjoy these recipes and create upon them.

I also bow deeply to all of my teachers.

One Love!

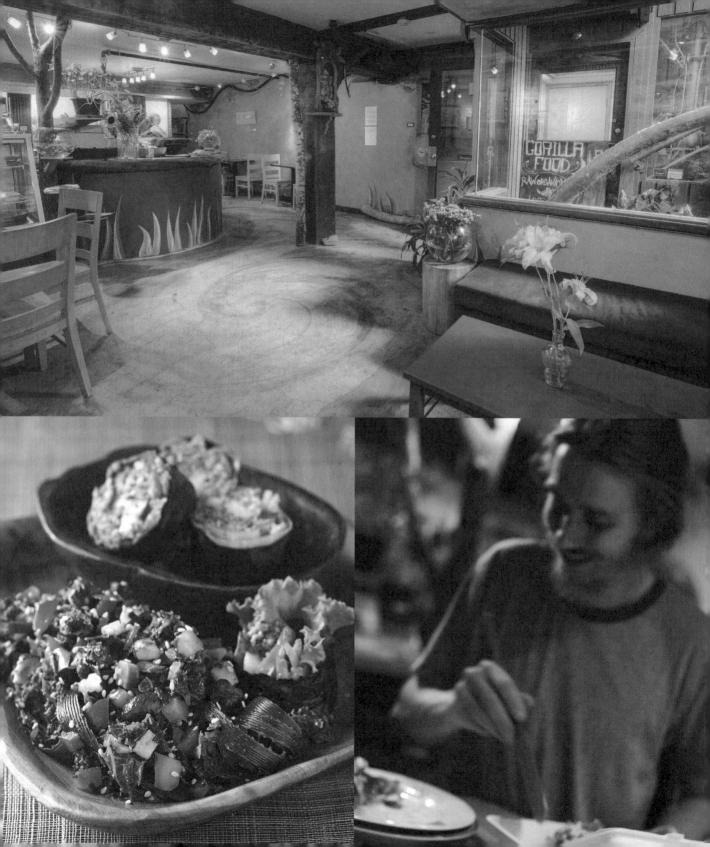

Introduction

As I've been compiling these recipes, it's allowed me to reflect on the times in which they were created and the experiences I've had with them. Going through my old recipe journals has reminded me of what I've learned, where I've been, all the great people I've met, and all that I've eaten on this journey of discovering these different foods.

The mission of Gorilla Food is to encourage and promote peace through food as well as through holistic supercharged health and nutrition, environmental and social activism, economics, arts, and culture. The idea for Gorilla Food, and my ambition to make it happen, started in 1996 when I was twenty years old and just discovering the great wide world of raw, vegan, and organic foods. At first, I was especially enthusiastic about the vibrancy of fresh-pressed juices and felt the whole world needed to know about their health benefits. I became eager to start a juice bar and to create a community hub for social interaction and for sharing holistic information. After years of travel, studies, experiences, and experiments, that idea for the small juice bar has come to be, and it's now blossomed into Gorilla Food, where we serve juices and so much more.

I feel blessed that I have been able to serve and learn from so many amazing people. I've gotten to do summer festival vending and travel to other countries to cater for various groups, yoga retreats, and individuals. I've worked in collaboration with friends on other cafés and restaurants. This service has been a joy and a journey!

It seems like both yesterday and a lifetime ago that I was jokingly calling it "Guerrilla Food" because, at first, when I couldn't afford to open a restaurant space, I served, catered, and delivered raw foods privately from an "underground" a.k.a. "guerrilla" kitchen. I would email weekly menus to customers, who could either have it delivered or pick up their orders themselves at the small garden-level suite of

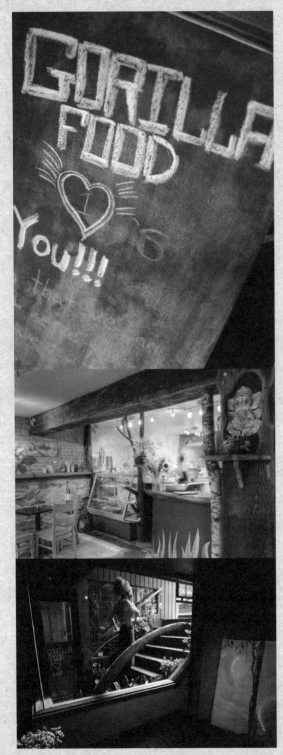

the house I had rented.

With the support of many amazing customers and through word-of-mouth, more people found out about it, and bit by bit it grew to become a small take-away window in the downtown core of Vancouver that in 2006 operated for two years. Then we moved to a larger sit-down space two doors away where we've been operating as a small café restaurant since 2007. There is an entire community of us working together to create the next phase of the Gorilla Food dream.

This book is a great part of that dream. Thank you for being a part of it!

I hope it will encourage you to discover the health benefits of the raw vegan lifestyle, and that you will enjoy making these recipes for yourself and for others. It has been such a joy creating these foods for our loyal customers over the past few years, singin' and dancin' in the kitchen all the while. And now it's my joy to share the Gorilla Food experience with you!

Gorilla Food: Organic, Vegan & Raw

Fresh, natural foods are what humans have always survived and thrived on. We used to eat only organic food—which was then known simply as "food." It's only in the last few generations that we have been eating foods that have been boxed, bagged, or canned; it is wiser and healthier for all of us that we eat only good, wholesome food that comes from the world's biggest produce supplier: Mother Earth and her mighty gardeners! Gorilla Food is part of a massive cultural shift toward fresh, natural, vegan foods.

Organic

This is the central foundation of Gorilla Food—we stand for organic food! We use only organic ingredients because of the clean and vital living and growing techniques used to cultivate them, resulting in produce that is healthier and better-tasting. Organic food is also often grown by really, really amazing people—I sometimes wonder if all the amazing organic farmers I know add magic to their crops, or if the amazing food they grow puts the magic into them!

I once read about a study conducted on gorillas in which zookeepers offered them both organic and non-organic bananas. The gorillas would first select the organic bananas and eat them with the peel on; when it came to the non-organic ones though, they would peel and discard the skin before eating them. Smart monkeys!

(Source: Organic Consumers Association: *organicconsumers.org/ Organic/bananas022403.cfm*)

To meet the highest organic food standards, certified growers and farmers must prove they follow sustainable food production methods—something we should all support! They pay attention to where their seeds come from, where their water comes from, what kind of inputs they add to the soil, and how close they are in proximity to toxins from other farms. They also often have a deep appreciation for Earth and how she sustains us. With every penny we spend on their products, we vote for our collective future; we are saying yes to the creation of peace and harmony and sustainability. Support local organic farmers to protect the future of our planet, our communities, and future generations to come. Go organic!

Which came first, the seed or the tree?

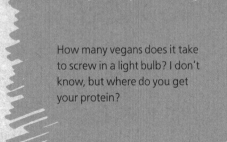

How many vegans does it take to screw in a light bulb? I don't know, but where do you get your protein?

Vegan

The word vegan comes from *vegetus*, a Latin word meaning "lively or vigorous." Vegan foods are derived from ingredients free from animal suffering. Veganism creates peace on many levels. The benefits to eating life-force-filled, organic, vegan, and raw foods are numerous:

• You will find yourself in a world surrounded by peace, energy, compassion, sustainability, and good flavors.

• You will be nourished with healthful, Earth- and animal-loving, cruelty-free food—and don't forget pesticide-free, fungicide-free, insecticide-free, synthetic-free, and radiation-free—food that is alive, colorful, beautiful, nutritious, and light-filled!

There is plenty of scientific evidence endorsing the advantages of eating a diet full of raw, organic fruits, veggies, seeds, and nuts. Organic, vegan, and raw foods are beneficial for the treatment of arthritis and fibromyalgia; they help to prevent diet-related cancers and cardiovascular disease, and play a role in preventing, treating, and even reversing type-2 (adult onset) diabetes, and they can be helpful for weight loss.

Eating fruits, vegetables, seeds, and nuts is one of the best ways to maintain an optimum point of health, feeding your body with an abundance of energy, phyto-nutrients, fiber, essential fats, proteins, vitamins, and whole-food synergy.

Raw

If many elements of foods and their nutritional qualities (for example, enzyme activity, oils, minerals, vitamins, and other phytonutrients) are destroyed by air, oxygen, and light, how about blasting them with intense heat and molecular manipulation from modern-day ovens, stoves, or microwaves? What does that do?

Gorilla Food's raw food cuisine is made from plant-based food ingredients kept in their most lively, whole, natural state. The raw and living food culinary art form generally allows for food processing and heating up to a point of 117°F (47°C). This is the temperature considered to be a heat threshold, preventing excessive damage to nutrients.

I've heard it said that every plant is a medicine for something, whether the healing quality comes from its beauty, flower, smell, root, bark, leaf, or seed. Plants, in their many varieties, forms, and preparations, assist with the holistic well-being of our physical, mental, and emotional health. Gorilla Food believes in medicinal plant food cuisine: fresh, simple, and real.

Living foods

A part of raw foods cuisine is the living food aspect, which focuses on our food being alive, growing, and feeding us life-force, which comes from sprouting seeds, nuts, and grains; culturing fruits or veg-gies; making nut and seed cheezes; and making fermented drinks like rejuvelac, kombucha, kefir, and wine.

Many people claim to feel cleaner and clearer in mind and body from eating living foods. Personally, I feel more con-nected to Earth and reality ... something that I've heard termed the "Gaia matrix"; I think it's "the Force." Environmental bonus points: we could afford to feed everyone on the planet if all our diets were plant-based. In the true raw foods diet, there is no packaging and no waste—and no energy is needed to cook.

> "Until he extends the circle of his compassion to all living things, man will not himself find peace."
> —Albert Schweitzer,
> French philosopher, physician, and musician
> (Nobel Peace Prize, 1952)

I often wonder if the violence we inflict on animals desensitizes us to it, or does it reflect the violence we cause ourselves and our human family? Are we so barbaric that we can kill an animal, steal her babies, and steal her milk and drink it or ferment it and eat it on a sandwich for lunch as if no harm has been done? Some of us profit from this, some of us pay for this to be done.

"As long as men massacre animals, they will kill each other. Indeed, he who sows the seeds of murder and pain cannot reap the joy of love."
—Pythagoras

"My refusing to eat flesh occasioned an inconveniency, and I was frequently chided for my singularity, but, with this lighter repast, I made the greater progress, for greater clearness of head and quicker comprehension. Flesh eating is unprovoked murder."
—Benjamin Franklin

"The greatness of a nation and its moral progress can be judged by the way its animals are treated."
—Mahatma Gandhi

International Ital

Ital derives from the word "vital," but begins with "I" to signify the unity of the speaker with all of nature. Ital cuisine is believed, in the Rastafari movement, to connect us with nature. There are different interpretations of Ital regarding specific foods. The general principle is that food should be natural or pure, and from the earth.

Many followers of the Ital diet are strict vegans because they believe humans are naturally vegetarian (based on human physiology and anatomy). They do not consider dairy products natural for human consumption (and many do not eat salt as well). Many Rastafarians believe that we all share Livity, or life energy. The intent of an Ital diet is to increase Livity. Ital is based in part on the belief that meat is dead, and consuming it would therefore work against Livity.

Give thanks for Livity!

To the kitchen

Here are a few tips to set up your kitchen right, some techniques that will give you a head-start with your new equipment, and some basic ingredients for your fridge and pantry.

Tools

Properly setting up your kitchen is the best way to support yourself if you want to integrate organic, vegan, raw foods into your life. Have fun as we go over the different tools that you may want to acquire.

1. Food Processor

Although I use a blender more often, a food processor is the first tool that I would take if I had to choose just one machine for the desert island. It can do almost all of what a blender can do, and more. (You can find a food processor in any department store and most kitchen stores. If you want to recycle or are on a budget, you might be able to pick one up at a thrift shop or yard sale.)

Varying size capacities, qualities, and powers are what differentiate the wide array of manufacturers or models. Each include different attachments that allow for varied thicknesses in slicing or different shreds and shapes. Usually there will be an s-blade (named after its shape), a slicing disc, and a shredding (grating) disc. The s-blade attachment can be used for purée-ing, chopping, and blending. The different disc attachments are great for shredding and slicing larger amounts of ingredients and allow us to work faster than we can with our hands.

2. Blender

The blender is used almost as much as the food processor. There is a large variance in quality between brands and types of blenders; the higher powered ones create creamier and smoother textures than the average department-store blender.

I like one brand, the Vita-Mix, best because, in addition to its super power, it has a tamper stick. This is a wand that allows you to stir your ingredients while the machine is running and not have to worry about getting a spoon or scraper caught in the dangerously high-speed blade.

3. Dehydrator

Dehydrators are pretty basic and can even be made at home. I've seen several home-built models that work great. Solar dehydrators are a good option too. The dehydrator helps to create raw and live-food versions of breads, cookies, crisps, and candies. You can also wilt foods by drying them for just a little while, so that when you marinate veggies or fruits, they will draw in more of the moisture and the flavors of the marinade.

With the dehydrator, you can create varying textures and forms by evaporating moisture from foods. For the sake of art or display, you can sculpt and shape these healing foods while they dry.

A dehydrator is similar to an oven, except that it can be regulated to a much lower temperature. Similar to baking, the machine evaporates water out of food, but much more slowly. (It can take between 12 and 96 hours instead of 45 minutes to 3 hours in an oven at higher temperatures.) A dehydrator is basically a box with shelves to hold mesh-bottomed trays. It has a heat source and a fan that moves the air out, blowing away the evaporating moisture from the food.

When I first started making more raw foods, I didn't have a proper dehydrator, so I would turn my gas oven to the lowest temperature (which was 150°F [66°C]) and hold the door open with a wide metal spoon. This was dangerous, but it allowed me to do my first sprouted-bread experiments. Things were much safer once I got an electric dehydrator!

It is best to dehydrate most food items on the mesh screens because they allow maximum air flow and will help to dry them out quickly. When dehydrating thin batters, you can use parchment paper (which should be thrown away after each use) or you can use the non-stick ParaFlexx sheets that come with the Excalibur dehydrator.

The advantage to the Excalibur brand is that it has a fan at the back that allows for an even airflow over all the trays. Some models have a fan at the bottom of the unit and blow from underneath, which means the trays have to be switched from top to bottom to achieve evenly dried food.

4. Juicers

A juicer separates the fiber from the water (or juice) of fruits, herbs, or vegetables. There are different styles of juicers that separate these properties in different ways. When purchasing a juicer, there are several things to think about: How good is the quality of the juice it produces? How easy is the juicer to clean? How much juice is left in the pulp? How loud is it? How expensive is it?

Some juicers will seem expensive, but they are worth the investment if you consider the increased quantity of juice you can obtain by not throwing away still-wet pulp. This is something you trade off with the cheaper, lower-quality juicers.

Some juicers are better for different types of fruits or veggies. Centrifugal

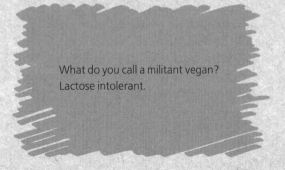

What do you call a militant vegan?
Lactose intolerant.

juicers are the cheapest to buy. They are easy to clean, juice roots and firm fruits well, but do not do green leaves at all. They are also usually the loudest of the juicers and the juice has a faster oxidization rate.

A hydraulic press will give you the most juice per weight of produce with the driest pulp. It will also give you the highest quality juice because, by pressing the produce, you are not exposing it to as much air as the spinning centrifugal-style juicer. However, the press is slower: it is a two-stage process consisting of first shredding the produce and then placing it in a cloth to filter the juice out with a high-pressure squeeze.

Augur-style juicers are mid-range in price, easy to clean, and quiet. They do all fruits, veggies, and leafy greens well. They are either horizontal or vertical and have a corkscrew augur that first draws the plant in, then squeezes it through the channel, forcing the juice through a screen and separating out the pulp.

The Green Star twin-gear juicer is the best all-round juicer for me because it does everything very well, including fruits, veggies, leafy greens, nut butters, and sorbets. The two-gear system shreds and squeezes the juice through a metal screen and the pulp out the other end into a catcher.

A citrus juicer can come in manual or electric, and be used both as a press or a reamer.

Note: The sooner you drink juice after juicing it, the better, because it will quickly deteriorate and become oxidized.

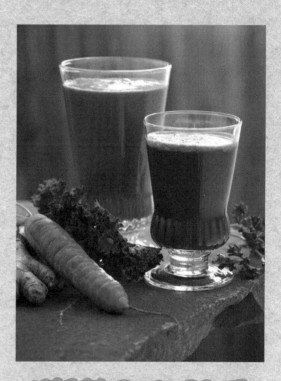

Why did the chicken cross the road? Because Colonel Sanders was chasing him.

5. Spirooli slicer

This is a great tool to have when preparing foods to replace pasta. There are a few brands similar to the Spirooli slicers; they all turn firm veggies, roots, and fruits into long strands that resemble spaghetti, fettuccini, or linguini noodles. We call these "New"dles.

6. Mandoline

This is a very useful tool, but be careful, it can also be very dangerous! A mandoline can cut an almost infinite variety of shapes and sizes of produce. It can help process quite a lot of food in a short amount of time, too, and without too much clean-up.

7. Knives

A chef's knife or two are great for basic chopping, dicing, mincing, and all-round use. Paring knives allow for more precision cuts or peeling, carving, and cleaning small blemishes or bruises on fruits and veggies. A serrated knife can be handy to have too, to make certain cuts.

8. Other good tools:

• A coffee grinder is great for pulverizing seeds, nuts, spices, and dry herbs. I have not found a better tool for powdering cacao nibs.

• Measuring spoons and measuring cups for both liquid and dry ingredients.

• Springform pans are really good for making raw pies.

• A thermometer so you can determine what the 117°F (47°C) threshold temperature feels like.

• A veggie peeler for cleaning fruits and veggies that can also be used for shaping them or making shavings, which are great for salads or as garnish.

• Flippers, turners, scrapers, spoons, spreaders, mixing bowls, and microplanes are also useful aids to creative food prep.

"Vegetarian food leaves a deep impression on our nature. If the whole world adopts vegetarianism, it can change the destiny of humankind."
—Albert Einstein

9. Water filter

There are many considerations when it comes to water. If you are going to go to all the effort of optimizing your diet, then you should consider filtering your water at the tap to remove chlorine and other harmful elements.

While the best source of water is spring water, bubbling fresh, cold, and straight from deep in the ground, it's not always available. I like to use a carbon-block water filter to remove the wide array of unwanted elements such as synthetic chemicals, bacteria, viruses, and pharmaceuticals that cycle through municipal tap water.

Make a point to connect with your local water source. This is another way to embrace Earth's universal energy grid!

Ingredients

This is what the dishes are made of—it's what it's all about! If you start out with great ingredients, you'll end up with great food. The ones I use in this book are not out of the ordinary; I've purposely chosen ingredients that are easily available. Farmers' markets and health food stores are stocked with amazing raw food staples. They are the best places to shop! When choosing ingredients, consider:

• Their backstory: Where did these ingredients come from? Who grew them? Why?

• What are their medicinal properties? What are their flavors?

• What different textures can be created from them?

• What season is it? What is ripe now?

• What does my body want? What do my guests want?

• What colors are right?

"Now I can look at you in peace; I don't eat you anymore!"
—Franz Kafka, while admiring fish in an aquarium

The five flavors are spicy, sweet, salty, sour, and bitter. Mixing different flavors is a good way to ensure that your diet has variety. Strengthen each flavor to match or contrast with another. If you experiment with different combinations, it will lead to many joyful meals!

This is a list of ingredients that will be used in the recipes to help you shop at the market and stock up your pantry.

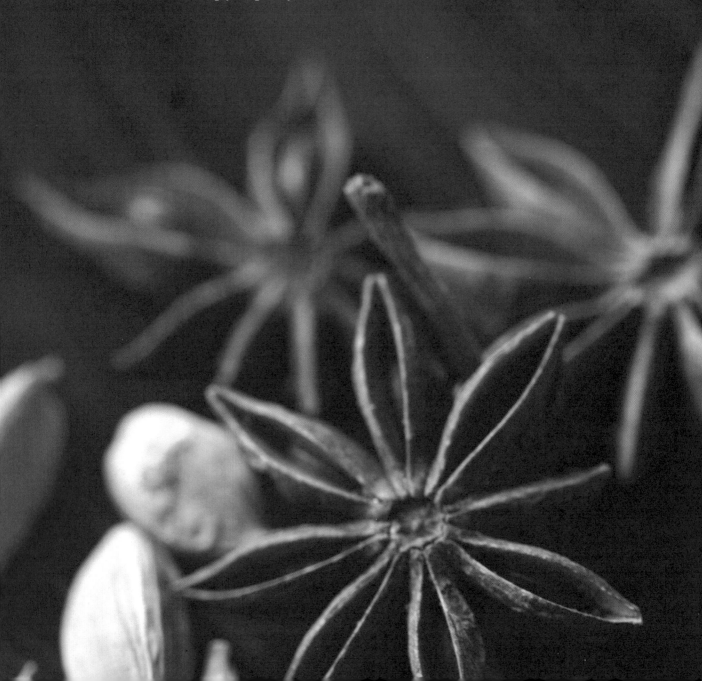

Fresh produce:

Apples
Avocados
Bananas
Basil
Beets: red or yellow
Blackberries
Broccoli
Burdock
Cabbage: purple or green
Carrots
Cauliflower
Celery
Chard
Cilantro
Collard greens
Cucumber
Daikon
Dandelion greens
Dates
Garlic
Ginger
Kale: green, lacinato,
   Siberian, etc.
Lemons
Lettuce: green leaf or
   romaine
Onions, yellow
Orange juice/oranges
Parsley: green, curly
Parsnips
Peppers, bell
Pineapple
Radishes
Spinach
Sprouts: alfalfa, clover,
   sunflower, etc.
Squash: butternut,
   kabocha, red kuri, etc.
Sunchokes
Strawberries
Tomatoes
Watercress
Zucchini

Oils and vinegar:

Apple cider vinegar
Cacao butter
Coconut oil
Flax seed oil
Olive oil
Sesame oil

Nuts:

Almonds
Brazil nuts
Cashews
Hazelnuts
Macadamia nuts
Pecans
Pistachios
Walnuts

Seeds:

Chia seeds
Buckwheat
Flax seeds
Hemp protein powder
Hemp seeds
Quinoa: white or red
Peanuts
Pine nuts
Pumpkin seeds
Sesame seeds
Sunflower seeds

Dried fruits:

Coconut flakes
Dried cherries
Goji berries
Golden berries
Mangos
Olives, sun-dried black
Pineapple
Raisins
Sun-dried tomatoes

Seaweeds and algaes:

Dulse
Nori sheets
Sea palm fronds
Spirulina
Wakame

Superfoods, spices, and dry herbs:

Açaí berry powder
Allspice
Astragalus
Bay leaves
Black pepper
Cacao nibs, powder,
   or paste
Camu camu powder
Caraway seeds
Cardamom
Carob
Cayenne pepper
Chamomile
Chili powder
Cinnamon
Cloves, whole or powdered
Coriander, ground
Cumin, ground
Curry powder
Fennel seeds
Ginger powder
Italian herbs, dried
   (parsley, basil, oregano,
   rosemary)
Juniper berries
Maca powder
Nutmeg, whole or ground
Paprika
Peppermint
Rooibos
Rosehips
Salt: Himalayan
Sarsaparilla root
St. John's Wort
Star anise pods, whole
Stevia
Turmeric powder
Vanilla powder

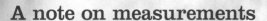

A note on measurements

At the restaurant, we use a scale for many of the recipes (so we can be precise with measurements), but since most people in North America do not have scales handy at home, we have rounded ingredients up or down a little on certain measurements. You are encouraged to experiment with the flavors of the recipes and make them your own.

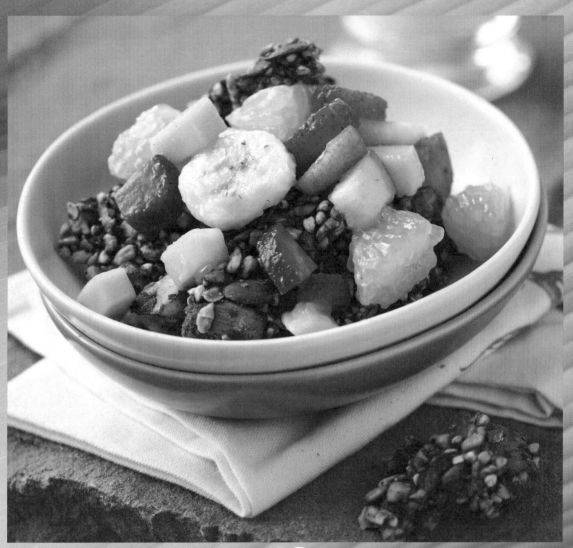

Breakfasts

Pre-soak

Brazilian Blackberry Grawnola

There are many antioxidants in this particularly purple breakfast. While staying in a cabin on a cold and damp West Coast island, I really enjoyed pouring warm water over the grawnola to soften and warm it. When dehydrating, I test it to see when the almonds and cashews are fully crunchy and dry; then I know it's done.

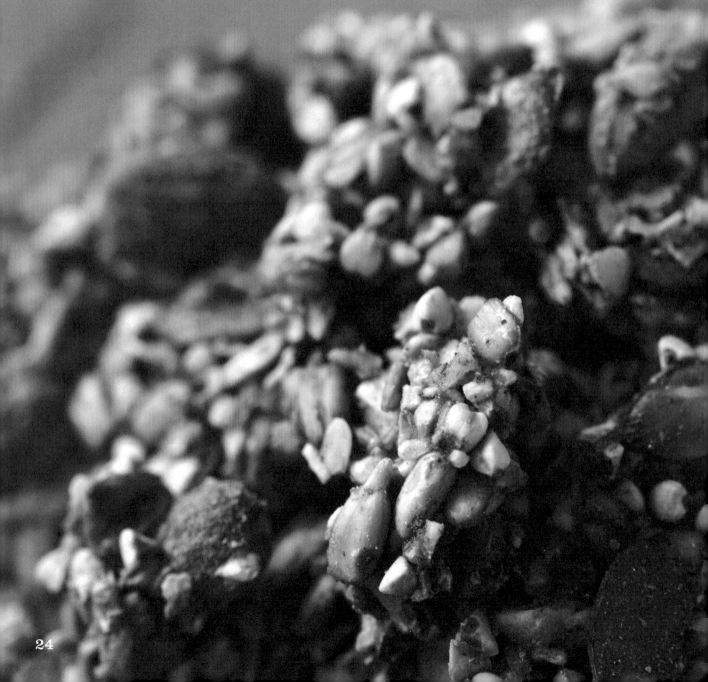

2 cups (500 mL) buckwheat
1½ cups (375 mL) sunflower seeds
¾ cup (185 mL) almonds
½ cup (125 mL) pumpkin seeds
⅜ cup (90 mL) cashews
3 cups (750 mL) Brazil nuts

½ cup (125 mL) goji berries
11 dates, pitted
3 bananas
2½ cups (625 mL) blackberries
1¼ cups (310 mL) blueberries
1 tbsp açaí berry powder

1. In a large bowl, soak buckwheat, sunflower seeds, almonds, and pumpkin seeds together overnight and rinse well before using.

2. In another bowl, soak cashews separately overnight and rinse well before using.

3. In a third bowl, soak Brazil nuts separately overnight and rinse well before using.

4. In the morning, in a small bowl, cover goji berries in water for approximately 1 hour to plump them up and hydrate them.

5. In a food processor with an s-blade, process Brazil nuts to a fine flaky consistency and then add to a large mixing bowl with all other rinsed seeds and nuts.

6. Drain goji berries and add them to the seeds and nuts.

7. In a food processor with an s-blade, blend dates, bananas, blackberries, blueberries, and açaí berry powder into a smooth sauciness and add to the nut and seed mix, stirring together thoroughly.

8. Spread the mix onto ParaFlexx sheets and dehydrate at 108°F (42°C) for 8–12 hours or overnight.

9. Flip over onto mesh sheets and continue to dehydrate at the same temperature for 2–3 more days until almonds and cashews are fully crunchy and dry.

Makes 6 cups (1½ L)

Cinnamon Apple Grawnola

I love eating this in a bowl with sliced bananas, apples, and berries—and with a Strawberry Bliss Up! Shake (p. 235) poured over top.

2 cups (500 mL) buckwheat
1½ cups (375 mL) sunflower seeds
¾ cup (185 mL) almonds
½ cup (125 mL) pumpkin seeds
½ cup (125 mL) cashews
¾ cup (185 mL) Brazil nuts
¾ cup (185 mL) coconut flakes

15 dates, pitted
2 tbsp hemp protein powder
1 tbsp ground cinnamon
1 tbsp maca powder
1 tsp vanilla powder
½ tsp salt
2 apples, cored

1. In a large bowl, soak buckwheat, sunflower seeds, almonds, and pumpkin seeds together overnight and rinse well before using.

2. In a separate bowl, soak cashews overnight and rinse well before using.

3. In another bowl, soak Brazil nuts overnight and rinse well before using.

4. In a food processor with an s-blade, chop Brazil nuts to a medium fine consistency and add to other nuts and seeds, including cashews.

5. Add coconut flakes to the mix.

6. In a food processor with an s-blade, process dates, hemp protein, cinnamon, maca, vanilla, salt, and apples to a smooth sauciness and then add to the seed and nut mix. By hand, stir together thoroughly.

7. Spread a ½-in (1-cm) thick layer of the mix on ParaFlexx sheets and dehydrate at 108°F (42°C) for 8–12 hours or overnight.

8. Flip over onto mesh sheets to continue to dehydrate at the same temperature for 2–3 more days, until the almonds and cashews are crunchy.

Makes about 9 cups (2⅛ L).

Clove & Orange Zest Grawnola

 Pre-soak

I like to have banana and pear slices with vanilla-infused almond (or hemp) sylk (p. 238 or 239) with this filling start to the day.

2 cups (500 mL) buckwheat
½ cup (125 mL) almonds
⅓ cup (80 mL) pumpkin seeds
1 cup (250 mL) sunflower seeds
⅓ cup (80 mL) quinoa
¼ cup (60 mL) chopped dried apricots
⅔ cup (160 mL) raisins
¼ cup (60 mL) goji berries

7 dates, pitted
1 tbsp hemp protein powder
1 tsp orange zest
1 tsp maca powder
¾ tsp ground cinnamon
¼ tsp salt
1 pinch ground cloves

1. In a large bowl, soak buckwheat, almonds, and pumpkin and sunflower seeds together overnight, and rinse well before using.

2. In a separate bowl, soak quinoa for 4–6 hours in water and rinse well before using. Add to rinsed buckwheat mixture.

3. In another bowl, cover and soak apricots, raisins, and goji berries in water for 1–3 hours, and drain before using. Reserve the sweet soaking water.

4. In a large bowl, combine soaked fruits with buckwheat, seeds, and nuts.

5. In a food processor with an s-blade, process dates, hemp protein, orange zest, maca powder, cinnamon, salt, and cloves into a smooth paste. Add soaking water, as needed, to thin out the paste. Pour into bowl with seed, fruit, and nut mix, and mix together well.

6. Spread wet grawnola on ParaFlexx sheets and dehydrate at 108°F (42°C) overnight. Flip over onto mesh sheets to dehydrate at the same temperature for another 2–3 days.

Makes 6 cups (1½ L) per sheet.

Fruit Salad with Cashews, Hemp Seeds & Hemp Seed Nogurt

This is super cleansing, hydrating, and full of vitamins! During my first summers as a vegetarian, my meals must have been eighty percent fruit salad.

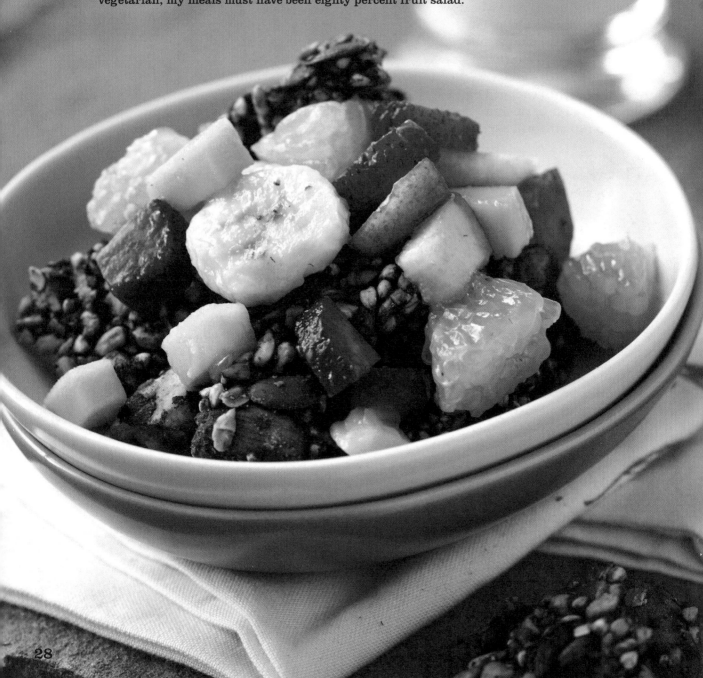

1 apple, cored and chopped

1–2 bananas, sliced

1 pear, cored and chopped

½ cup (125 mL) sliced strawberries

⅓–½ cup (80–125 mL) peeled and chopped citrus (orange, grapefruit, pomelo, etc.)

⅓–½ cup (80–125 mL) mixed berries (blackberries, blueberries, Saskatoon berries, etc.)

1–2 cups (250–500 mL) chopped seasonal fruit (peaches, nectarines, kiwis, plums, etc.)

½ cup (125 mL) cashews

⅓ cup (80 mL) hemp seeds

1 tbsp lemon juice

⅓–½ cup (80–125 mL) Hemp Seed Nogurt (p. 92)

1. In a bowl, toss fruits with cashews, hemp seeds, and lemon juice.

2. Serve with Hemp Seed Nogurt on the side or drizzled over top.

Makes 2 servings.

Walnut & Banana Pancakes

Pancakes are an instant portal into childhood for me. My grandpa, Jim, was the main breakfast chef around the summer cabin. He was always ready at the griddle, set to make more orders for the kids. Unfortunately, these aren't the kind of pancakes you can wake up and spontaneously decide to make! Serve with your choice of Sweet Creams (p. 92-93) and/or Fruit Compotes (p. 95).

1½ cups (375 mL) buckwheat
1 cup (250 mL) sunflower seeds
1 tbsp flax seeds
2 apples, cored and chopped
6 bananas, sliced

1¼ tbsp ground cinnamon
¼ tsp salt
2 tbsp coconut flakes
½ cup (125 mL) chopped walnuts

1. Soak buckwheat and sunflower seeds overnight or for at least 6 hours, rinsing well before using.

2. In a blender or coffee grinder, grind flax seeds to a powder and set aside in a bowl.

3. In a food processor with an s-blade, process buckwheat and sunflower seeds to a creamy peanut butter consistency. Pour into a bowl.

4. In a food processor, process apples, bananas, cinnamon, and salt to a purée and add to the bowl.

5. Add the ground flax seeds, coconut flakes, and walnuts to the dough, and mix everything thoroughly by hand.

6. On ParaFlexx sheets, form round pancakes by hand (4 per sheet) and dehydrate them at 108°F (42°C) for 8–12 hours. Flip over the pancakes onto mesh sheets and continue to dehydrate at the same temperature for another 4–8 hours, until the outside is dry but the inside is still moist.

Makes 7–8 pancakes.

Morning Curry Crêpes

You can actually have these crêpes any time of the day, but they make a great late breakfast on a slow and easy weekend. The spices will get you charged and feeling blessed for the day! Plate with a serving of Basic Greens (p. 120) drizzled with Citrus Mint Dressing (p. 72) or any other dressing you like.

1 Ginger Tomato Crêpe (p. 54)
¾ cup (185 mL) Curry Veggies (p. 165)
2–3 tbsp Green Coconut Curry
  Dressing (p. 73)

¼ cup (60 mL) Guacamole (p. 78)
⅔ cup (160 mL) sprouts (alfalfa, clover,
  radish, sunflower, etc.)

1. Place Curry Veggies in center of crêpe.

2. Drizzle with Green Coconut Curry Dressing.

3. Drizzle with Guacamole.

4. Fill with sprouts.

5. Fold the bottom of the crêpe up toward the top. Then fold the two sides in toward each other, and roll up the crêpe. Lay on a plate with flaps down.

Makes 1 serving (multiply ingredients to serve more).

Breakfast Burrito

This is a great bite at any time of the day. Experiment with different salad fillings or savory goos. You could serve this with a bed of Basic Greens (p. 120) and a side of Hemp Seed Nogurt (p. 92) for dipping or dressing.

1 Celery Basil Crêpe (p. 53)
⅓ cup (80 mL) Dilly Brazilly Creme (p. 89)
1 cup (250 mL) Tossed and Tenderized Deep Greens (p. 134)

3 tbsp Super-Food Dressing (p. 74)
2 tbsp chopped Chili Almonds (p. 56)
½ avocado, sliced
¾ cup (185 mL) sprouts (alfalfa, clover, radish, sunflower, etc.)

1. In center of crêpe, spread a generous strip of Dilly Brazilly Creme.

2. In a mixing bowl, toss the Tossed and Tenderized Deep Greens and Super-Food Dressing together.

3. Mound the dressed Deep Greens in center of crêpe.

4. Sprinkle crushed Chili Almonds over Deep Greens.

5. Layer with avocado slices.

6. Top with sprouts.

7. Fold the bottom of the crêpe up toward the top. Then fold the two sides in toward each other, and roll up the burrito. Lay on a plate flaps down.

Makes 1 serving (multiply ingredients to serve more).

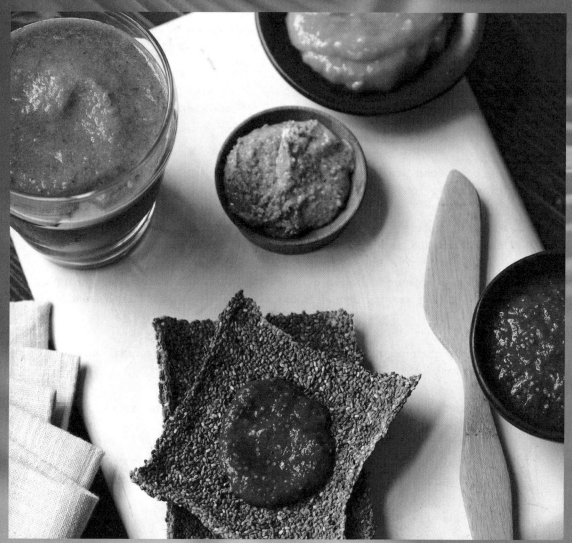

Breads, Crackers, Crêpes & Nuts

Brazil Nut & Olive Crusty Bread

I'm happy for this creation! The coconut flour gives it the feel of shortbread in the mouth.

3 cups (750 mL) Brazil nuts
1½ medium zucchinis, chopped
1 sweet bell pepper, chopped
1 cup (250 mL) chopped parsley

2 tbsp lemon juice
1¼ cups (310 mL) coconut flour
¾ cup (185 mL) pitted sun-dried black
  olives

1. In a bowl, soak Brazil nuts overnight or for at least 12 hours and rinse well before using. Reserve 1 cup of soaking water.

2. In a food processor with an s-blade, purée zucchinis, bell pepper, parsley, and lemon juice to a paste. Set aside in a bowl.

3. In a food processor with an s-blade, blend Brazil nuts to a paste, adding a bit of the soaking water if needed to keep the mix from sticking to the sides of the processor.

4. Add coconut flour and 2 cups water to the nuts and blend until smooth. Add to puréed veggies.

5. Chop olives coarsely and then add them to the veggie and nuts in the mixing bowl. Mix well by hand.

6. Spread mixture (about ¼–½-in [½–1-cm] thick) on ParaFlexx sheets and mark bread slices with the dull side of a knife (around 4 crackers x 4 crackers).

7. Dehydrate at 108°F (42°C) for 8–12 hours or overnight.

8. Flip over onto mesh sheets and continue to dehydrate at the same temperature for about 36 hours or until completely dry.

Makes 16 crackers.

Veggie Flax Bread

With this recipe idea I was originally aiming to create a flax tortilla, but it didn't turn out that way after all. Instead, it became a mainstay sandwich on the Gorilla Food menu.

¼ cup (60 mL) sun-dried tomatoes
2 cups (500 mL) water
3½ cups (830 mL) whole flax seeds
1½ cups (375 mL) chopped onions

6–8 celery stalks
1 tbsp hemp protein powder
1 tsp salt
3 tbsp olive oil

1. In a bowl, soak sun-dried tomatoes in 2 cups of water overnight or for at least 1 hour. Reserve 1½ cups (375 mL) soaking water.

2. In a blender or coffee grinder, grind the flax seeds into powder. Set aside in a bowl.

3. In a food processor with a shredding disc, shred half the onions and half the celery. Add to ground flax seeds.

4. In a food processor with an s-blade, purée the sun-dried tomatoes and remaining onions, celery, hemp protein, and salt.

5. Pour in olive oil and slowly add sun-dried tomato soaking water to thin mixture. Pour into ground flax seeds and, using your hands, squeeze the mix thoroughly to create a sticky dough.

6. Spread evenly about ¼-in (½-cm) thick on ParaFlexx sheets and cut into 4 even-sized slices per sheet.

7. Dehydrate at 108°F (42°C) for 8–16 hours.

8. Flip over onto mesh sheets and continue to dehydrate at the same temperature for approximately 3 hours or until the top has crusted over, but bread is still moist.

Makes 8 slices.

Curry Squash Bread

One day I came back to Gorilla Food with a large food processor that we had been saving up for, and I was itching to try it out. The weekend before at the farmers' market, some beautiful squash had caught my eye, and I had no plans for it yet, so I came up with this recipe. It was a winner right away. The trick is keeping it moist: flip it over as early as possible and monitor it often.

½ cup (125 mL) buckwheat
⅓ cup (80 mL) dried mango
½ cup (125 mL) whole flax seeds (for grinding)
2 cups (500 mL) chopped winter squash (butternut, kabocha, hubbard, etc.)

½ sweet bell pepper, cut into 1-in (2½-cm) pieces
½ medium zucchini, cut into 1-in (2½-cm) pieces
⅔ tsp salt
1 tbsp curry powder
1 pinch ground cayenne
⅓ cup (80 mL) whole flax

1. In a bowl, soak buckwheat overnight or for at least 6 hours and rinse well before using.

2. In a bowl, soak dried mango for ½–2 hours and rinse well before using.

3. In a blender or coffee grinder, grind ½ cup flax seeds. Set aside.

4. In a food processor with an s-blade, purée drained, soaked mango.

5. Add rinsed buckwheat to the mango purée and blend to a creamy peanut butter consistency. Set aside.

6. In a food processor with an s-blade, purée squash, bell pepper, zucchini, salt, and spices.

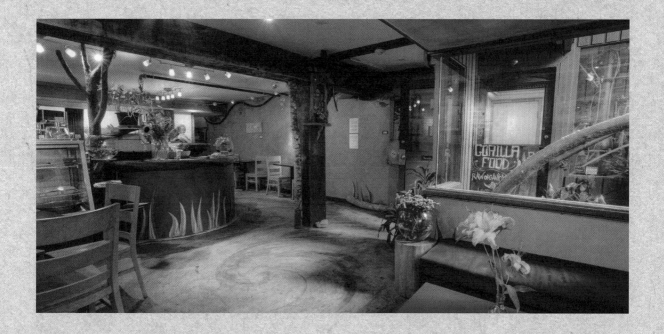

7. Add the buckwheat mix and whole and ground flax seeds to the squash purée. Process further until well mixed.

8. Spread the mix about ¼-in (½-cm) thick on 2 ParaFlexx sheets and cut into 4 even slices per sheet.

9. Dehydrate at 108°F (42°C) for 8–12 hours or overnight.

10. Flip over onto mesh sheets and continue to dehydrate until the top has crusted over, but bread is still moist.

Makes 8 slices.

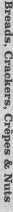

Breads, Crackers, Crêpes & Nuts

Pre-soak

Strawberry, Goji, Chia & Flax Bread

You gotta love strawberry season; there are so many to eat even when your belly is full!

2 tbsp goji berries

¾ cup (185 mL) goji berries (to mix
  with raisins)

¼ cup (60 mL) raisins

⅓ cup (80 mL) hazelnuts

2 cups (500 mL) whole flax seeds

1 cup (250 mL) chia seeds

⅓ apple

2 bananas

5 cups (1¼ L) sliced strawberries

⅛ tsp ground nutmeg

¾ tsp ground cinnamon

½ tsp mesquite powder

1. In a bowl, cover and soak 2 tbsp goji berries in water for 1–2 hours.

2. In another bowl, cover and soak ¾ cup goji berries and raisins in water for 1–2 hours. Reserve ⅝ cup (150 mL) soaking water.

3. In another bowl, cover and soak hazelnuts in water for 1–2 hours and rinse before using.

4. In a blender or coffee grinder, grind flax seeds into a powder. Set aside in a large bowl.

5. Chop hazelnuts into coarse but small pieces and add to ground flax seeds.

6. Stir chia seeds into flax and nuts.

7. In a food processor with an s-blade, purée 2 tbsp goji berries, raisin and goji soaking water, apple, bananas, strawberries, nutmeg, cinnamon, and mesquite. Add to flax.

8. Add the ¾ cup goji berries and raisins and combine all ingredients thoroughly.

9. Spread dough evenly, about ¼-in (½-cm) thick, on ParaFlexx sheets and cut into 4 even-sized slices per sheet.

10. Dehydrate at 108°F (42°C) for 8–12 hours or overnight.

11. Flip over onto mesh sheets and continue to dehydrate at the same temperature until the top has crusted over, but bread is still moist.

Makes 8 slices.

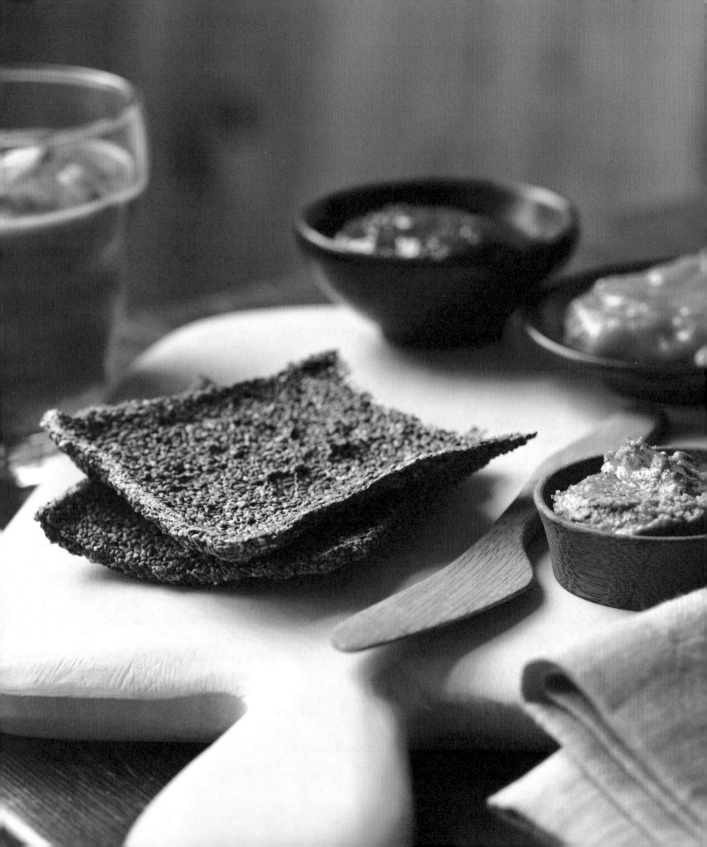

Chia Toast

With its subtle flavor, this light but dense seed crisp makes great toast to put toppings on.

5 cups (1¼ L) chia seeds
2½ bananas
1 tsp lemon juice
¾ tsp salt

1. In a bowl, soak chia seeds in 12 cups (3 L) water for 1–3 hours.

2. With a fork or a potato masher, mash bananas with lemon juice and salt. When smooth, combine thoroughly with chia seeds.

3. Spread mix ¼–½-in (½–1-cm) thick on Paraflexx sheets and score with the dull side of a knife, 3 crackers wide by 3 crackers high.

4. Dehydrate at 108°F (42°C) for 12–16 hours.

5. Flip over onto mesh sheets and continue to dehydrate at the same temperature for another 24 hours or until completely dry.

Makes 9 crackers.

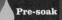 **Pre-soak**

Chia Sea Crisps

A super simple-to-make, dense, and nutritious seed crisp that you can snack on anytime, use as the base of an open-faced sandwich, or break into pieces to serve canapés on.

½ cup (125 mL) sliced wakame seaweed
1¾ cups (415 mL) chia seeds
4 cups (1 L) water
¼ tsp salt

1. In a bowl, mix all ingredients together and let sit for 3 hours.

2. Spread the mixture about ½-in (1-cm) thick on ParaFlexx sheets and dehydrate at 108°F (42°C) overnight or for 8–12 hours.

3. Flip over onto mesh sheet and continue to dehydrate at the same temperature for an additional 12–24 hours, or until fully dry and crispy.

4. Break into random pieces or carefully break or cut the sheet into squares or rectangles.

Makes 1 sheet (number of crisps will vary).

Cinnamon Apple Flax Crackers

I love the subtle sweetness of these crackers. I've always had a fondness for cinnamon raisin toast, and these remind me of it!

⅜ cup (90 mL) sesame seeds
1 cup (250 mL) sunflower seeds
4 cups (1 L) flax seeds
1⅓ cups (315 mL) raisins

1 cup (250 mL) raisins
11 dates, pitted
⅜ tsp ground cinnamon
3 apples, cored

1. In a bowl, soak sesame seeds and sunflower seeds overnight or for at least 6 hours. Rinse well before using.

2. In a separate bowl, soak flax seeds for 4–6 hours.

3. In two separate bowls, soak each portion of raisins for 2–4 hours.

4. To the bowl with flax seeds, add rinsed sunflower and sesame seeds and 1⅓ cup (315 mL) raisins.

5. In a food processor with an s-blade, purée 1 cup raisins, dates, cinnamon, and apples. Pour into the seeds and mix thoroughly.

6. Spread seed mix about ¼-in (½-cm) thick on ParaFlexx sheets and, with the dull side of a knife, mark 18 cracker shapes per sheet.

7. Dehydrate at 108°F (42°C) for 12–16 hours.

8. Flip over onto mesh sheets and continue to dehydrate at the same temperature for another 36–48 hours.

Makes 54 crackers.

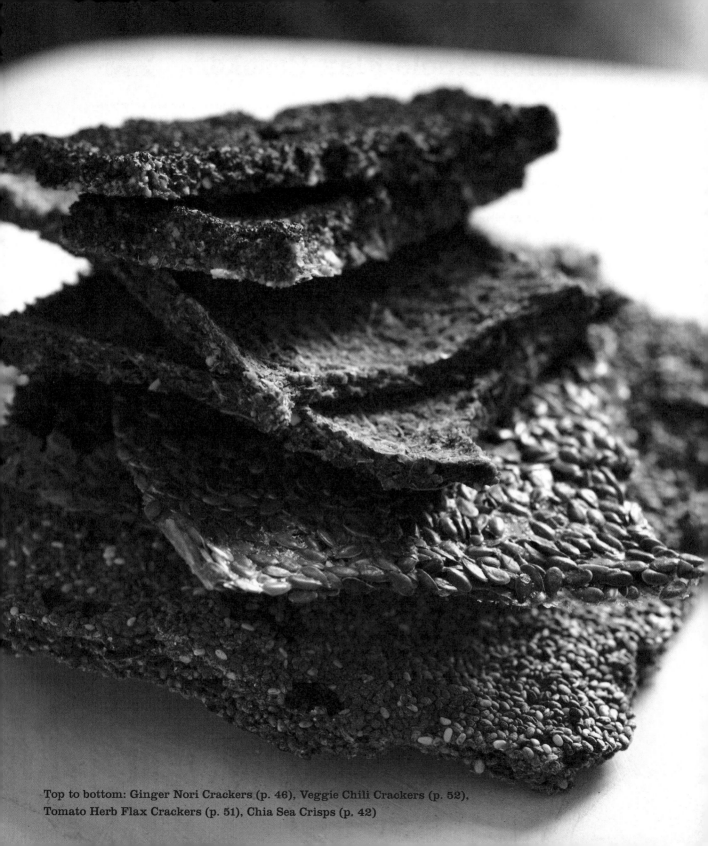

Top to bottom: Ginger Nori Crackers (p. 46), Veggie Chili Crackers (p. 52), Tomato Herb Flax Crackers (p. 51), Chia Sea Crisps (p. 42)

Eastern Bunny Crackers

I created these eastern-spiced crackers just before Easter one year while packing up for a long weekend. This is an example of how dehydrating can be a great way to preserve an abundance (or excess!) of food.

½ cup (125 mL) pumpkin seeds
½ cup (125 mL) Tahini (p. 69)
1 cup (250 mL) chopped cauliflower
¾ cup (185 mL) chopped tomatoes
2 tbsp lemon juice
½ tsp ground cumin
¼ tsp ground cayenne

¼ tsp ground turmeric
¼ tsp black pepper
½ tsp salt
¾ medium zucchini
½ sweet bell pepper
1 medium carrot

1. In a bowl, soak pumpkin seeds for 4 hours and rinse well before using.

2. In a food processor with an s-blade, purée all ingredients except zucchini, bell pepper, and carrot. Empty into a bowl.

3. In a food processor with a shredding disc, shred zucchini, bell pepper, and carrot. Add to the bowl with other ingredients and mix to combine well.

4. Spread batter about ¼-in (½-cm) thick on ParaFlexx sheets and, with the dull side of a knife, mark 18 cracker shapes per sheet.

5. Dehydrate at 108°F (42°C) for 8–12 hours or overnight.

6. Flip over onto mesh sheets and continue to dehydrate at the same temperature for another 12–24 hours or until crispy.

Makes 18 crackers.

Breads, Crackers, Crêpes & Nuts

Ginger Nori Crackers

These might be my favorite crackers. Even though they're Asian-inspired, they're great with Guacamole (p. 78).

4 cups (1 L) Sunny Ginger Pâté (recipe below)
1 raw sheet of nori seaweed

1. Spread Sunny Ginger Pâté about ¼–½-in (½–1-cm) thick on ParaFlexx sheets and, with the dull side of a knife, mark 18 cracker shapes per sheet.

2. Blend nori sheet in a blender (using the tamper) until powdered. Sprinkle 1 tbsp of nori powder onto the batter.

3. Dehydrate at 108°F (42°C) for 10–13 hours.

4. Flip onto mesh sheets and continue to dehydrate at the same temperature for another 30 hours.

Makes 18 crackers.

 Pre-soak ## Sunny Ginger Pâté

3½ cups (830 mL) sunflower seeds
1¼ cups (310 mL) raisins
1 cup (250 mL) chopped ginger
5 garlic cloves
1½ zucchinis, roughly chopped
6 carrots, roughly chopped
1½ tsp salt

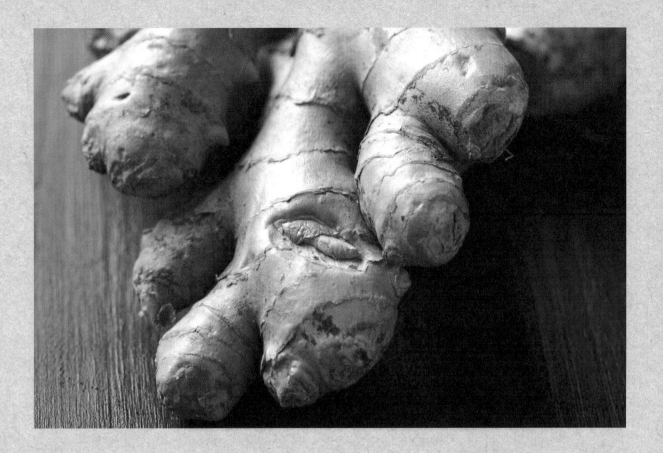

1. In a bowl, soak seeds overnight or for at least 6 hours and rinse well before using.

2. In a separate bowl, soak raisins for 20–60 minutes.

3. In a food processor with an s-blade, mince ginger and garlic. Add zucchinis, carrots, and salt, and process until finely minced. Empty into a large bowl.

4. In a food processor with an s-blade, purée raisins and add to veggie mix.

5. In a food processor, process rinsed seeds into a paste. Add them to veggie mix and mix everything very well by hand.

Makes 4 cups (1 L).

Sesame & Walnut Pesto Crackers

This is a great way to preserve produce, such as the last of your basil, at the end of the summer gardening season.

6 cups (1½ L) walnuts
1 cup (250 mL) Tahini (p. 78)
1 garlic clove
4 cups (1 L) fresh basil leaves
3 cups (750 mL) chopped sweet bell peppers
1 cup (250 mL) chopped sunchokes

2½ cups (625 mL) chopped tomatoes
4 large or 7 small kale leaves, chopped
1 medium zucchini, chopped
¾ tsp salt

1. In a bowl, soak walnuts for 4 hours or overnight and rinse well before using.

2. In a food processor with an s-blade, process walnuts into a paste. Add to a bowl with Tahini.

3. In a food processor with an s-blade, mince garlic. Add rest of ingredients and purée. Add to walnut and Tahini and mix to combine well.

4. Spread across ParaFlexx sheets and, with the dull side of a knife, mark 18 cracker shapes per sheet.

5. Dehydrate at 108°F (42°C) for 12–16 hours.

6. Flip over onto mesh sheets and continue to dehydrate at the same temperature for another 24–30 hours until crispy.

Makes 36 crackers.

Tomato Ginger Crax

You can serve these as the base to an appetizer (see p. 101), with a salad, or use them to scoop a dip (see pp. 75-82).

2 cups (500 mL) sunflower seeds
1½ cups (375 mL) almonds
1¼ cup (310 mL) raisins
1 cup (250 mL) chopped ginger
5 garlic cloves
8 cups (2 L) chopped kale

1½ zucchinis, roughly chopped
1 stalk celery, chopped
6 carrots, roughly chopped
1¾ tsp salt
2 cups (500 mL) chopped
  tomatoes

1. In a bowl, soak seeds and almonds overnight or for at least 6 hours and rinse well before using.

2. In a separate bowl, soak raisins for around 20 minutes–1 hour.

3. In a food processor with an s-blade, mince ginger and garlic. Add the kale, zucchini, celery, carrots, and salt, and process until all are finely minced. Add tomatoes and continue until puréed. Pour into a large bowl.

4. In a food processor with an s-blade, purée raisins and add to the veggie mix.

5. In a food processor, process rinsed seeds and almonds to nearly a paste consistency. Add them to veggie mix. Combine ingredients until well-mixed.

6. Spread the batter about ¼-in (½-cm) thick to the edges of ParaFlexx sheets and, with the dull side of a knife, mark 18 cracker shapes per sheet.

7. Dehydrate at 108°F (42°C) for 12–18 hours.

8. Flip over onto mesh sheets and continue to dehydrate at the same temperature for another 24 hours or until crispy.

Makes 36 crackers.

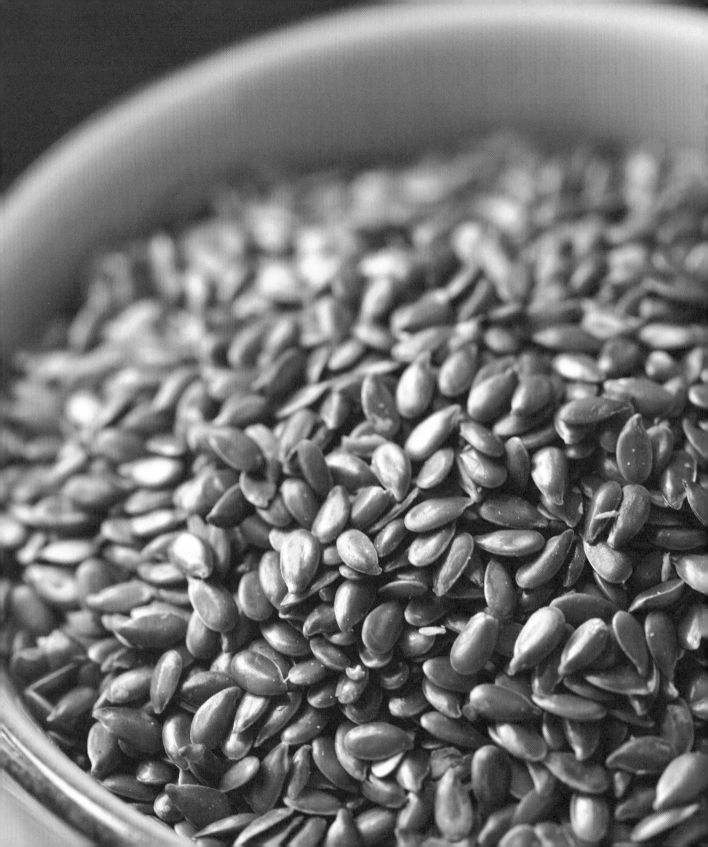

Tomato Herb Flax Crackers

I remember how amazed I was by the texture of soaked flax seeds when I first learned how to make flax crackers. There are endless flavor possibilities. Much better than a bag of fried potato chips!

6 cups (1½ L) flax seeds
6 cups (1½ L) water
4 cups (1 L) Ital Herb Tomato Sauce (p. 66)
1½ tsp salt

1. In a bowl, soak flax seeds in water for 4–6 hours, until all the water is absorbed.

2. Add Tomato Sauce and salt and mix to combine well.

3. Spread flax mix ¼-in (½-cm) thick on ParaFlexx sheets and, with the dull side of a knife, mark 16 cracker shapes per sheet.

4. Dehydrate at 108°F (42°C) for about 12 hours.

5. Flip onto mesh sheets and continue to dehydrate at the same temperature for another 24 hours or until completely dry.

Makes 32 crackers.

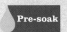

Veggie Chili Crackers

Dehydrated crackers keep well if they are dried completely. Make plenty in advance so you'll always have some on hand.

½ cup (125 mL) buckwheat
3 cups (750 mL) sunflower seeds
1⅓ cups (310 mL) flax seeds
5 cups (1 1/4 L) chopped kale
5 cups (1 1/4 L) chopped collards
4–5 carrots, chopped

½ red bell pepper, chopped
3 celery stalks, chopped
1½ medium zucchinis, chopped
2½ tsp salt
1 tbsp ground chili seasoning
½–¾ tsp ground cayenne

1. In a bowl, soak buckwheat and sunflower seeds in water overnight or for at least 6 hours and rinse well before using.

2. In coffee grinder or blender, grind flax seeds to a powder.

3. In food processor with s-blade, purée kale, collards, carrots, peppers, celery, and zucchini. Empty pulpy mix into a bowl.

4. In food processor, blend buckwheat and sunflower seeds with salt and spices into a creamy peanut butter consistency. Add to veggie mix.

5. Add ground flax and combine well.

6. Spread mix ¼-in (½-cm) thick on ParaFlexx sheets and score crackers with the dull side of a knife (4 crackers wide by 4 crackers high).

7. Dehydrate at 108°F (42°C) for about 12 hours.

8. Flip over onto mesh sheets and continue to dehydrate at the same temperature for another 36 hours or until completely dry.

Makes 32 crackers.

Celery Basil Crêpes

Here's a raw savory crêpe (or tortilla) that can be filled with veggies and sauces to mimic a burrito. You can also use it to wrap up a salad or as an eating utensil for other dishes, such as the Great Gorilla salad (p. 132).

1½–2 medium carrots, chopped
1 celery stalk, chopped
2 tbsp Hemp Seed Basil Pesto (p. 80)
⅔ cup (160 mL) chopped avocado

2 tbsp lemon juice
½ tsp salt
1 cup (250 mL) water

1. In a blender, purée all ingredients.

2. Pour onto ParaFlexx sheets and spread into two circles, each about ¼-in (½-cm) thick. Dehydrate at 108°F (42°C) for 8–16 hours.

Makes 2 crêpes.

Savory Tomato Crêpes

You can fill these crêpes with an endless variety of fillings; try spreading with Olive Tapenade (p. 76) and filling with sprouts and Basic Greens (p. 120) tossed in Lemon Herb Flax Dressing (p. 73). They are great at any time of day.

2 cups (500 mL) Ital Herb Tomato
  Sauce (p. 66)
3 tbsp ground flax seeds

⅔ cup (160 mL) Guacamole
  (p. 78)

1. In a blender, purée all ingredients until smooth.

2. Pour onto ParaFlexx sheets and spread into two circles about ¼-in (½-cm) thick. Dehydrate at 108°F (42°C) for 8–16 hours.

Makes 2 crêpes.

Ginger Tomato Crêpes

This started out as a drying experiment at the restaurant that went into the dehydrator the day before a one-day holiday. We returned the next day to a new pliable texture to work with. You can fill these crêpes with an endless number of ingredients!

½ cup (125 mL) sun-dried tomatoes
⅛ garlic clove
¾-in (2-cm) piece ginger
1 tbsp chopped onions
1 cup (250 mL) chopped tomatoes

½ tsp salt
1 date, pitted
2 tbsp flax seeds
½ cup (125 mL) chopped avocado

1. Cover and soak sun-dried tomatoes in water for at least 2 hours. Reserve 1 cup (250 mL) of soaking water.

2. In a blender, blend all ingredients plus 1 cup (250 mL) soaking water until smooth.

3. Pour onto ParaFlexx sheets and spread into two circle about ¼-in (½-cm) thick. Dehydrate at 108°F (42°C) for 8–16 hours.

Makes 2 crêpes.

Tomato Sesame Crêpes

These crêpes are delicate and have a nice flavor. Fill them with Basic Greens (p. 120) tossed with your choice of dressing.

2 cups (500 mL) chopped tomatoes
2 tbsp lemon juice
¼ tsp salt
3 tbsp sesame seeds

½ tsp ground cayenne
½ head lettuce (romaine, curly green leaf, curly red leaf, etc.)

1. In a blender, purée all ingredients until smooth.

2. Pour onto ParaFlexx sheets and spread into two circles about ¼-in (½-cm) thick. Dehydrate at 108°F (42°C) for 8–16 hours.

Makes 2 crêpes.

Breakfast Nuts

I can't believe it's not maple! You've got to make lots of these, because it's hard to not eat them all before they're ready.

2 cups (500 mL) pecans
1 cup (250 mL) walnuts
2 bananas
1 tsp ground cinnamon
⅜ tsp salt
3 dates, pitted
1 tsp maca powder

1. In a bowl, soak pecans and walnuts together for 4 hours or overnight and rinse well before using.

2. In a food processor with an s-blade, process bananas, cinnamon, salt, dates, and maca powder until puréed.

3. In a bowl, blend nuts with purée until well-mixed.

4. Spread coated nuts on ParaFlexx sheets and dehydrate at 108°F (42°C) for about 3 days or until crispy.

5. Once dried, break into segments.

Makes 3 cups (750 mL).

Chili Almonds

A super great snack or crunchy addition to any dish. When I first started the Gorilla Food take-away window (a very small space with limited dehydrator capacity), I had two customers who would buy all of the Chili Almonds whenever they could—whoever got there first. We couldn't keep up, as they take so long (5 days!) to fully dry. I suggest making them in big batches!

4 cups (1 L) almonds
⅜ cup (90 mL) chopped onions
2–3 garlic cloves
3 tbsp chopped shallots
13 dates, pitted

1 tsp ground cayenne or
 Thai chilies
2½ tsp salt
½–1 cup (125–250 mL) lemon
 juice

1. In a bowl, soak almonds overnight and rinse well before using.

2. In the food processor with an s-blade, process all ingredients except almonds to a smooth paste. Pour paste onto rinsed almonds and mix thoroughly.

3. Spread coated almonds on ParaFlexx sheets, one or two almonds thick, and dehydrate at 108°F (42°C) for 8 hours or overnight.

4. Flip almonds over into a bowl, break them up by hand, and place on mesh sheets. Continue to dehydrate at the same temperature for about 4 more days or until they are crunchy and fully dry.

Makes 4–4½ cups (1–1⅛ L).

Chilly Dill Willy Pistachios Pre-soak

These are another one of my most favorite snacks ever!

3 cups (750 mL) pistachios
⅜ cup (90 mL) pistachios
3–4 sprigs fresh dill
⅓ clove garlic
¼ medium zucchini, chopped
⅔ sweet bell pepper, chopped
1 tsp salt
⅜ tsp ground cayenne
4 tbsp lemon juice

1. In a bowl, soak 3 cups (750 mL) pistachios overnight or for at least 5 hours and rinse well before using. Place into a bowl.

2. In a food processor with an s-blade, blend rest of ingredients to a paste and pour over the pistachios. Toss to mix well.

3. Spread coated pistachios on ParaFlexx sheets and dehydrate at 108°F (42°C) for 8 hours or overnight.

4. Spread on mesh sheets and continue to dehydrate at the same temperature for 2–3 days or until crunchy.

Makes about 3¼ cups (810 mL).

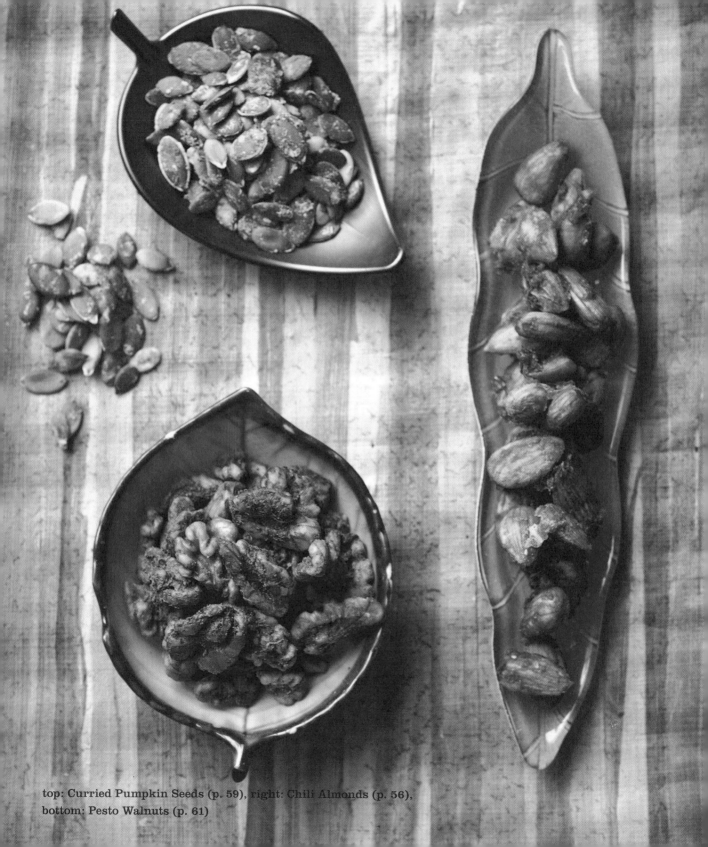

top: Curried Pumpkin Seeds (p. 59), right: Chili Almonds (p. 56),
bottom: Pesto Walnuts (p. 61)

Curried Pumpkin Seeds

These are good as a snack on their own or as a topping for salads or savory dishes such as the Rawmein "New"dles (p. 148).

2½ cups (625 mL) pumpkin seeds
1 carrot, chopped
1–2 kale leaves
½ tsp salt
2 tsp curry powder
1 pinch cayenne chili powder
2 tsp lemon juice
⅓ cup (80 mL) orange juice
¼ sweet bell pepper
1 tbsp water

1. In a bowl, soak pumpkin seeds overnight or for at least 4 hours, and rinse well before using. Place in a bowl.

2. In a blender, add rest of ingredients and blend until smooth. Pour over pumpkin seeds and mix thoroughly.

3. Spread coated seeds thinly and evenly on ParaFlexx sheets and dehydrate at 108°F (42°C) for 8 hours or overnight. Spread on mesh sheets and continue to dehydrate at the same temperature for 3 more days or until dry.

Makes 2½ cups (625 mL).

Chunky Monkey Trail Mix

A huge bag of this mix once got me through a three-week surfing trip when I didn't have much access to food.

1½ cups (375 mL) cashews
1 cup (250 mL) Brazil nuts
¾ cup (185 mL) pistachios
⅔ cup 160 mL) pecans
¾ cup (185 mL) sunflower seeds
½ cup (125 mL) walnuts
¾ cup (185 mL) almonds

9 dates, pitted
1 tbsp cacao powder, for rolling
  dates in
1⅓ cups (315 mL) raisins
½ cup (125 mL) goji berries
1¼ tsp ground cinnamon
1 cup (250 mL) cacao nibs

1. In a bowl, soak cashews overnight or for at least 4 hours and rinse well before using.

2. In a separate bowl, soak Brazil nuts overnight and rinse well before using.

3. In a third bowl, soak all other seeds and nuts together overnight and rinse well before using.

4. Place all seeds and nuts on mesh sheets and dehydrate at 108°F (42°C) for 3–4 days until almonds and Brazil nuts are dry and crunchy.

5. Chop dates and roll in a dusting of cacao powder.

6. In a large mixing bowl, toss nuts, seeds, and dates with rest of ingredients until well-mixed.

Makes 9–10 cups (2¼–2½ L).

Pesto Walnuts Pre-soak

Sometimes I'll eat too many of these—but they're so good! They're delicious and densely packed with nutrition!

4 cups (1 L) walnuts
¾–1 cup (185–250 mL) Hemp Seed Basil Pesto (p. 80)
½ tsp salt

1. In a bowl, soak walnuts overnight or for at least 6 hours and rinse well before using.

2. Add Pesto and salt to walnuts and mix thoroughly.

3. Spread coated walnuts evenly on ParaFlexx sheets and dehydrate at 108°F (42°C) for 8 hours or overnight. Spread onto mesh sheets and continue to dehydrate at the same temperature for 3 more days or until dry.

Makes 4 cups (1 L).

Traveler's Mix

This is another good combination of fruits and nuts. It's amazing to learn about the nutritional qualities packed into each ingredient and what each is good for.

¾ cup (185 mL) cashews
⅓ cup (80 mL) Brazil nuts
1 cup (250 mL) almonds
⅓ cup (80 mL) sunflower seeds
⅓ cup (80 mL) pumpkin seeds

½ cup (125 mL) goji berries
½ cup (125 mL) mulberries
⅓ cup (80 mL) raisins
8 dates, pitted and chopped

1. In a bowl, soak cashews overnight or for at least 4 hours and rinse well before using.

2. In a separate bowl, soak Brazil nuts overnight and rinse well before using.

3. In a third bowl, soak almonds, sunflower seeds, and pumpkin seeds together overnight and rinse well before using.

4. Place seeds and nuts on mesh sheets and dehydrate at 108°F (42°C) for 3–4 days until almonds and Brazil nuts are dry and crunchy.

5. In a large mixing bowl toss nuts and seeds with rest of ingredients until well-mixed.

Makes 3½ cups (830 mL).

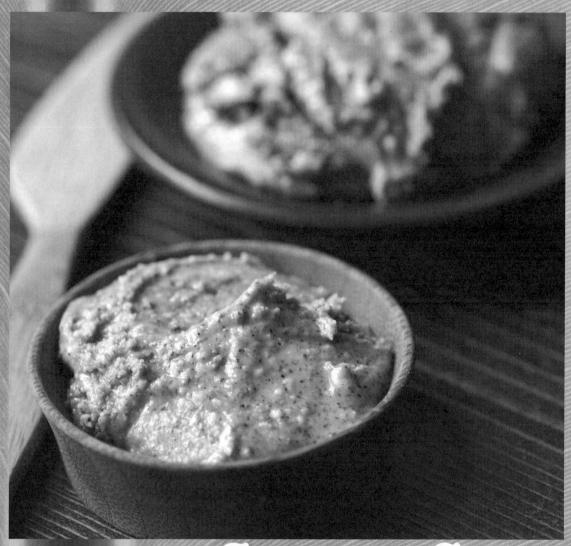

Sauces, Goos, Sweet Creams, Cheez & Spreads

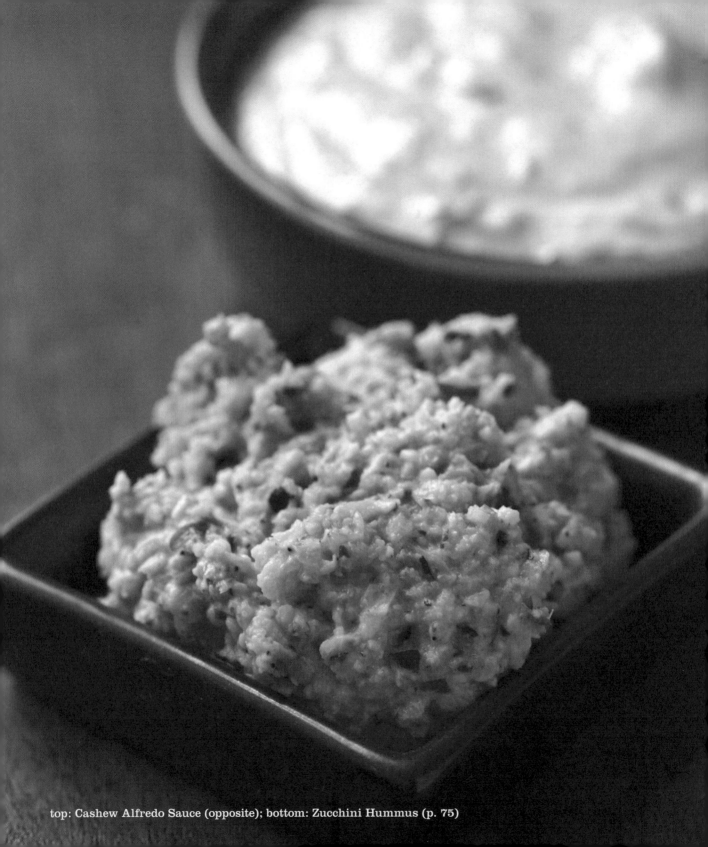

top: Cashew Alfredo Sauce (opposite); bottom: Zucchini Hummus (p. 75)

Cashew Alfredo Sauce

When I was sixteen, I started working in an Italian kitchen as a dishwasher. Learning how to make the Alfredo sauce was one of my first distractions. Thanks to cashews, I realized I didn't want to use dairy anymore. I could peacefully get all the oils and creaminess I wanted from different seeds or nuts instead of from animals. This sauce can be tossed with "New"dles to make vegan linguini and can be used in many other recipes.

1 cup (250 mL) cashews
½ garlic clove
1 tbsp lemon juice
⅛ tsp salt

⅛ tsp ground black pepper
½ cup (125 mL) water
¼ cup (60 mL) finely minced parsley

1. In a blender, purée all ingredients except parsley until creamy and smooth. Pour into a bowl and set aside.

2. In a bowl, add parsley to cashew cream and stir until well-mixed.

Makes 1¼–1½ cups (310–375 mL).

Green Cashew Coconut Curry Sauce

Thank goodness for Thai cuisine! It's been a staple that helped inspire my love for eating Ital. Spice it up a bit more or less depending on your preference. This one makes a great topping for the Delhi Doubler Burger (p. 160) and deliciously dresses the Curry Veggie Nice Bowl (p. 164).

⅔ cup (160 mL) chopped cilantro
⅝ cup (150 mL) coconut flakes
¼ cup (60 mL) cashews
½ tsp salt
2 tbsp lemon juice

½ garlic clove
1-in (2½-cm) piece ginger
½ tsp ground cayenne
½ cup (125 mL) water

1. In a blender, process all ingredients until smooth.

Makes 1 cup (250 mL).

Ital Herb Tomato Sauce

After making raw tomato sauces for the first time and seeing how easy it was, I wondered why I had been going through all of the trouble of stewing the tomatoes down. This was so much better and more refreshing. Serve with Lasagna-nanda (p. 146), Ital Veggie Pizza (p. 157), and much more.

¼ cup (60 mL) sun-dried tomatoes
1 garlic clove
½ celery stalk
2½ tsp dried mixed Italian herbs
  (parsley, basil, oregano, rosemary)
⅓ tsp salt
2½ cups (625 mL) chopped
  tomatoes

1. Soak sun-dried tomatoes in water overnight or for around 2 hours until soft.

2. In a food processor with an s-blade, mince garlic, celery, herbs, and salt.

3. Add drained sun-dried tomatoes and purée well. Pour into a large bowl and set aside.

4. In a food processor, process fresh tomatoes to a saucy and slightly chunky consistency. Add to sun-dried tomato paste and mix until well-combined.

Makes 3 cups (750 mL).

Nice 'n' Spicy Sesame Chili Sauce

This sauce reminds me of a certain boxed mac and cheese for some reason. It's way spicier and way better, though!

⅜ cup (90 mL) sesame seeds
¾ cup (185 mL) water
2 tbsp lemon juice

1 tsp salt
1½ tsp ground cayenne
⅜ cup (90 mL) sesame oil

1. In a blender, purée all ingredients except oil until creamy.

2. Add oil and blend just until smooth and incorporated.

Makes 1½ cups (375 mL).

Southern Fire Hot Sauce

Levels of spice tolerance, I've learned, vary a lot. It's a good example of how we all have our own perceptions and experiences of the same thing. Use this fiery sauce on Spicy Zucchini Chips (p. 108) or on a Southern Fire Veggie Burger (p. 163).

¾ cups (185 mL) chopped tomatoes
2 tbsp sesame seeds

¼ tsp salt
¼ tsp ground cayenne

1. In a blender, purée all ingredients until smooth.

Makes ¾ cup (185 mL).

Oh My Gado Peanut Sauce

Whenever I make this sauce, I think of my two good brothers, Rick and Long Life, both of whom enjoy making spicy peanut soup. You can use lime instead of lemon juice, or spice this up or down with more or less cayenne. Thin it out with twice the carrot juice and water to make what I call Selectah Sauce. Use on Peanut Selectah Pizza (p. 155) or in Oh My Gado-Gado Nice Bowl (p. 166)

½ cup (125 mL) jungle peanuts*
½ date, pitted
4–8 sprigs fresh cilantro
¼ tsp salt
⅛–¼ tsp cayenne chili powder

¼ cup (60 mL) carrot juice
2 tbsp water
¼-in (½-cm) piece ginger
2 tsp lemon juice

1. In a blender, purée all ingredients until smooth.

Makes 2–4 servings.

*Jungle peanuts are an heirloom strain of peanuts that come from Ecuador. They are a good source of protein and healthy oils. If not available, substitute regular raw peanuts.

Tahini Drizzle

This sauce was designed for the Falafel Wraps (p. 168) but it also goes nicely tossed with the Basic Greens (p. 120) or Tossed and Tenderized Deep Greens (p. 134).

⅓ cup (80 mL) sesame seeds
1½ tbsp lemon juice
⅔ cup (160 mL) water
⅛ tsp salt
⅓ tsp ground cumin

⅓ tsp ground paprika
½ date, pitted
1 pinch ground cayenne
¼ cup (60 mL) minced parsley

1. In a blender, purée all ingredients except parsley until smooth.

2. Stir parsley into the sauce.

Makes 1–1¼ cups (250–310 mL).

Tahini

This Middle Eastern staple has become a Western one, too. The sharper the food processor blade, the easier it is to break through the shells of the tiny sesame seeds.

3 cups (750 mL) sesame seeds

1. In a food processor with an s-blade, process seeds to a creamy consistency. If they heat up before finishing, place in the fridge to cool and then continue to process again until creamy.

Makes 3 cups (750 mL).

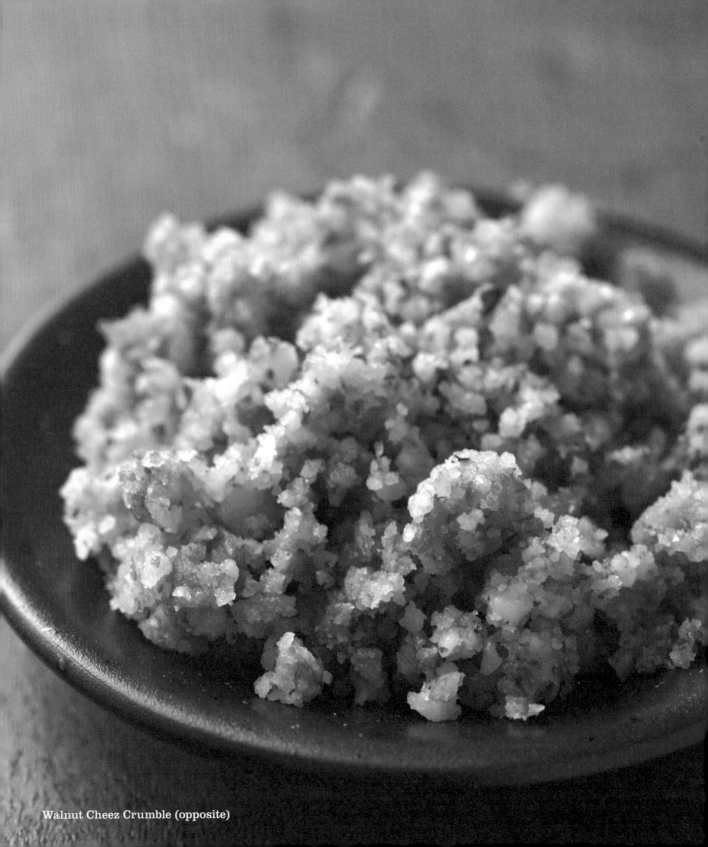

Walnut Cheez Crumble (opposite)

Walnut Cheez Crumble

It's so simple but so good! This originated as a pizza topping and came to find a home in a few other recipes after that. Toss it on any dish as a large component or simply use as a garnish.

1½ cups (375 mL) walnuts (for soaking)
1½ cups (375 mL) walnuts
2 tsp salt

1. In a bowl, soak 1½ cups walnuts for about 1 hour and rinse well before using.

2. In a food processor with an s-blade, pulse-process dry walnuts and salt with the soaked walnuts until crumbly.

Makes 2½–3 cups (625–750 mL).

Salty Mango Concoct

This is a good off-season replacement for fresh mango, or for when you're waiting for your mangos to ripen. It is used in the Ocean Wrap (p. 172) and the International Maki rolls (p. 171), and could also be served as a sweet accompaniment in a salad or on a veggie burger.

1 cup dried mango slices
¼ tsp salt

1. In a bowl, soak mangos for 2 hours in enough water to submerge.

2. In a food processor with an s-blade, process mangos and salt to a purée.

Makes ¾ cup (185 mL).

Citrus Mint Salad Dressing

Mmmmint—one of my favorite smells and flavors! Use on your choice of greens.

2 tbsp grapefruit juice
½ cup (125 mL) orange juice
2 tbsp lemon juice
2–3 sprigs fresh mint

¼ tsp salt
1 pinch ground cayenne
1½ tbsp flax oil
1½ tbsp olive oil

1. In a blender, process all ingredients to a smooth consistency.

Makes 1 cup (250 mL).

Ginger Avocado Dressing

This is a sweet creamy salad dressing that complements many different dishes such as the Cashew Alfredo Zucchini Linguini (p. 144) or Lasagna-nanda (p. 146).

½ cup (125 mL) orange juice
2 tsp finely chopped ginger
1 pinch salt

½ tbsp flax oil
½ avocado

1. In a blender, purée all ingredients until smooth and creamy.

Makes ¾ cup (185 mL).

Green Coconut Curry Dressing

This is good not only as a salad dressing, but also on a pizza or veggie burger; it can also be used as a soup base. Make it thicker (use less water) and you've got Green Coconut Curry Sauce.

¼ cup (60 mL) cilantro
¼ cup (60 mL) coconut flakes
¼ cup (60 mL) cashews
¼ tsp salt
1 tbsp lemon juice

¼–⅓ garlic clove
¼–⅓-in (6–8-mm) piece ginger
¼ tsp ground cayenne
⅜ cup (90 mL) water

1. In a blender, using the tamper, blend all ingredients until smooth.

Makes ¾–1 cup (185–250 mL).

Lemon Herb Flax Dressing

This is a light simple dressing to use when you want to fully appreciate the salad greens for their taste and texture. It is also good for marinating veggies.

3 tbsp lemon juice
3 tbsp Hemp Seed Basil Pesto (p. 80)
3 tbsp flax oil

3 tbsp olive oil
⅜ tsp salt
2 tbsp water

1. In a blender, process all ingredients until smooth and creamy.

Makes ⅞ cup (210 mL).

Super-Food Dressing

One of the great things about making your own dressings is that you can add nutritional supplements like super-food powders to them, as in this dressing.

⅓ cup (80 mL) cilantro
¼ cup (60 mL) lemon juice
2 tbsp parsley
½-in (1-cm) piece ginger
¼–⅓ avocado
1 cup (250 mL) water
1 tbsp hemp seeds
1 tbsp hemp protein powder

2 tbsp almonds
¼ tsp camu camu powder
2 tbsp goji berries
¼ tsp salt
1 pinch ground cayenne
¼ tsp spirulina
¼ tsp ground turmeric
¼ tsp açaí powder

1. In a blender, process all ingredients until smooth and creamy.

Makes 2 cups (500 mL).

Walnut Cilantro Dressing

I like to use this dressing on the Ital Veggie Pizza (p. 157) or over a bowl of Tossed and Tenderized Deep Greens (p. 134).

¾ cup (185 mL) walnuts
1 cup (250 mL) orange juice
⅓ cup (80 mL) chopped cilantro

¼ tsp salt
¼ medium zucchini, chopped

1. In a blender, process all ingredients until smooth and creamy.

Makes 2 cups (500 mL).

Zucchini Hummus

The first live hummus I ever made was with sprouted chickpeas. My stomach wasn't keen on the chickpeas, but I was into the tahini. The next time I made it, I tried to replace the chickpeas with soaked almonds, then zucchini, which I liked for its creaminess and mild flavor. This hummus is like the classic Middle Eastern version in its versatility: it can be used as a spread, dip, or dressing.

¾ cup (185 mL) sesame seeds
3 garlic cloves
⅓ cup (80 mL) coarsely chopped
  parsley
3½ tbsp lemon juice
⅓ tsp salt
1–1½ zucchinis, roughly chopped

1. In a food processor with an s-blade, process seeds until they reach the consistency of smooth peanut butter (tahini). Set aside in a bowl.

2. In a food processor, mince garlic with an s-blade.

3. Add parsley, lemon juice, salt, and zucchinis and blend until coarsely chopped.

4. Add tahini to food processor and blend all ingredients together until smooth and creamy.

Makes 2 cups (500 mL).

Basic Olive Tapenade

A super yummy, rich spread for crackers, breads, and sandwiches.

1½ garlic cloves
2 cups (500 mL) sun-dried black olives, pitted

1 pinch ground cayenne
2 tbsp olive oil

1. In a food processor with an s-blade, mince garlic.

2. Add olives, cayenne, and olive oil and process to a chunky texture.

Makes 1¾ cups (415 mL).

Monkey Tapenade

I can eat this in and on almost everything: veggie slices, crackers, breads, salads. It's one of my favorite flavors lately.

½ garlic clove
¼ cup (60 mL) chopped parsley
¼ red bell pepper
1 cup (250 mL) sun-dried black olives,
  pitted
1 pinch ground cayenne
1 tbsp olive oil
¼–⅓ cup (60–80 mL) Raisin Chutney (p. 81)

1. In a food processor with an s-blade, mince garlic.

2. Add parsley and bell peppers and mince.

3. Add olives, cayenne, olive oil, and Raisin Chutney and process to a spreadable paste, leaving just a bit of texture.

Makes 1⅓ cups (315 mL).

Guacamole

Every day is great when it has guacamole. Give thanks for all the avocado farmers in the world!

2–3 avocados
2 tbsp lemon juice
¼–⅓ tsp salt

1. In a bowl, mash together avocado, lemon juice, and salt with a fork or a potato masher until creamy.

Makes 1 cup (250 mL).

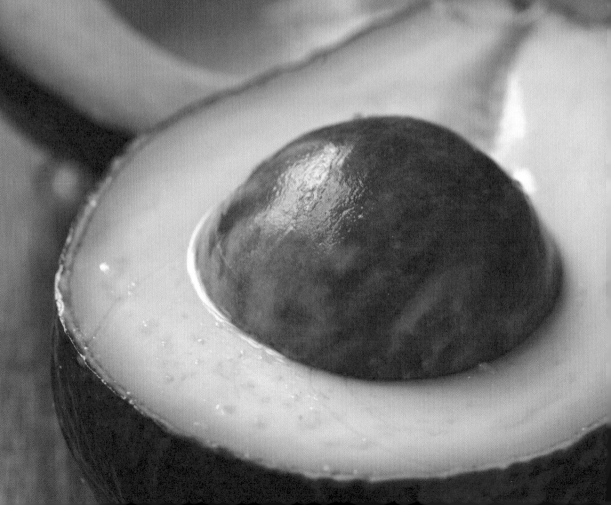

Salsa

The puréed date sweetens this just a bit—I'd say it's the secret to this salsa.

1 date, pitted
½ tsp salt
¼ tsp ground cayenne
3 tbsp lemon juice
½–⅔ cup (125–160 mL) chopped
   yellow onions
2 cups (500 mL) chopped tomatoes
½ cup (125 mL) minced cilantro

1. In a food processor with an s-blade, process date, salt, and cayenne, then slowly incorporate lemon juice to blend until smooth.

2. Add onions and tomatoes and pulse-process them into a chunky sauce (or chop or dice them by hand and add). Pour into a mixing bowl.

3. Stir cilantro into salsa and mix to combine well.

Makes 2½ cups (625 mL).

Hemp Seed Basil Pesto

I like to have pesto around for its great flavor and richness. It's nutritious and an excellent source of healthy fat. Use in Lemon Herb Flax Dressing (p. 73), Primo Pesto Wraps (p. 106), Kunda-Linguini Rising (p. 144) or simply tossed with "New"dles (p. 148).

1–2 garlic cloves
3 cups (750 mL) fresh basil leaves
½ cup (125 mL) walnuts
¼ tsp salt

2 tbsp hemp seeds
2 tbsp olive oil
2 tbsp lemon juice

1. In a food processor with an s-blade, mince garlic.

2. Add basil and process until finely minced.

3. Add rest of ingredients and process into a spreadable paste.

Makes 1 cup (250 mL).

Raisin Chutney Pre-soak

A version of one of my favorite sauces ever, made by Rick Letwinka, my bro and teacher. For a time I worked in his restaurant and on his farm, the Heliotrope in Regina, Saskatchewan.

1 cup (250 mL) raisins
¼ cup (60 mL) water
½ cup (125 mL) apple cider vinegar

¼ cup (60 mL) chopped fresh ginger
2 garlic cloves

1. In a bowl, soak raisins in water and apple cider vinegar for 1–4 hours.

2. In a food processor with an s-blade, purée all ingredients until smooth.

Makes 1¾ cups (415 mL).

Apple Chutney

This warming and fresh chutney is a good accompaniment to many different foods; try it with Curry Veggie Nice Bowl (p. 164) and don't miss it on Circa Loco Tops (p. 104) too.

1 apple, cored
⅛ tsp ground cumin
1 pinch ground coriander
⅛ tsp ground turmeric

1 pinch ground cloves
1 pinch ground dried ginger
⅛ tsp salt

1. In a food processor with an s-blade, pulse-process all ingredients until mix is still slightly chunky but nearly puréed.

Makes ½ cup (125 mL).

Pre-soak

Ocean Pâté

This pâté contains some excellent building blocks for the body. At Gorilla Food, we serve it in the Ocean Wrap (p. 172). It's really good served on a salad, too.

½ cup (125 mL) sunflower seeds
½ cup (125 mL) walnuts
4 celery stalks
1½ medium carrots

1 cup (250 mL) chopped dulse
¼ tsp spirulina
2 tbsp hemp seeds

1. In a bowl, soak sunflower seeds and walnuts for at least 6 hours or overnight and rinse well before using.

2. In a food processor with an s-blade, process soaked seeds and walnuts with rest of ingredients until the pâté is finely minced.

Makes 2 cups (500 mL).

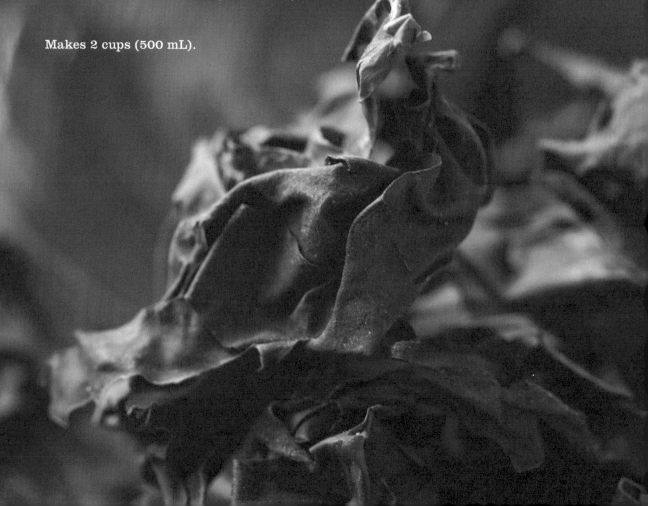

Fresh Ketchup

A classic to go with the burgers, 'cause what's a veggie burger without ketchup?!

¼ cup (60 mL) sun-dried tomatoes
⅛ garlic clove
¾-in (2-cm) piece ginger
1 tbsp chopped onions
⅛ tsp salt
½–1 date, pitted
1 cup (250 mL) chopped fresh tomatoes

1. In a blender, process all ingredients to a smooth consistency.

Makes 1 cup (250 mL).

Coconut Lemon Butter

David, one of Gorilla Food's great chefs, and I were preparing to cater a One Love, One Yoga event one night, and came up with this recipe at the last minute. It was much enjoyed and finished off the meal perfectly with the Circa Loco Tops (p. 104).

1 cups (250 mL) coconut flakes
1½ tbsp lemon juice
1 pinch salt
1 pinch ground cayenne
2–3 tbsp coconut oil

1. In a food processor with an s-blade, process all ingredients except for coconut oil until smooth.

2. Add coconut oil and mix until just combined.

Makes 1 cup (250 mL).

Thai Wrap Pâté

Pre-soak

Bless up Annie Jubb for teaching me to make seed pâté! This can be used in the Thai Fresh Wraps (p. 107), on a salad, or as a spread in a sandwich or on crackers.

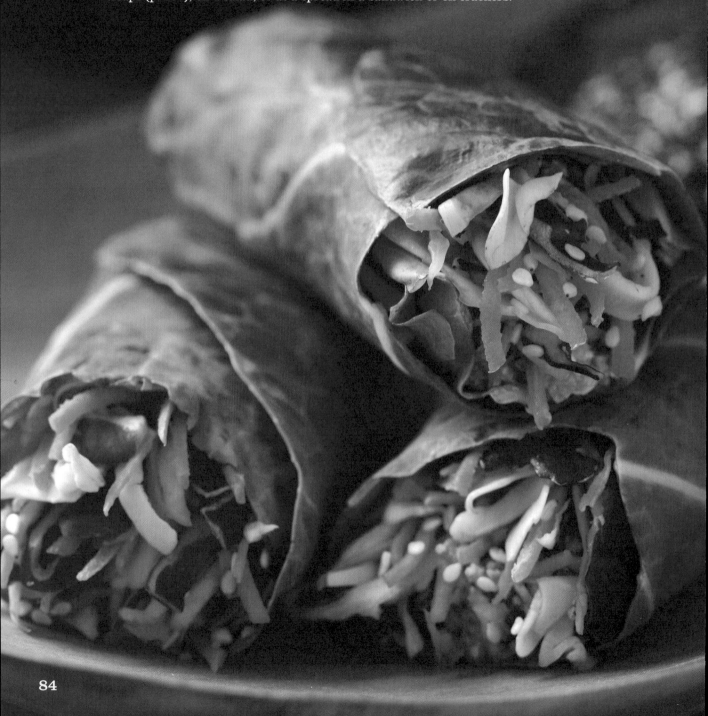

1 cup (250 mL) sunflower seeds
2 tbsp raisins
¼ garlic clove
¾–1 carrot, chopped
¼ medium zucchini, chopped

4 cups (1 L) kale and/or collards,
  chopped (you can use any leftover
  stems and leaves from preparing the
  wrappers for the Thai Fresh Wrap
  [p. 107])
¼ tsp salt

1. In a bowl, soak seeds for at least 6 hours or overnight and rinse well before using.

2. In a separate bowl, soak raisins for 2 hours or overnight in the fridge.

3. In the food processor with an s-blade, process seeds until crumbly but a bit sticky. Place in a bowl.

4. In a food processor with an s-blade, mince garlic. Add carrot, zucchini, kale/collards, and salt, and process until smooth. Add to seeds.

5. In a food processor with an s-blade, purée raisins. Add to veggie and seed mix and combined until well-mixed.

Makes 1½ cups (375 mL).

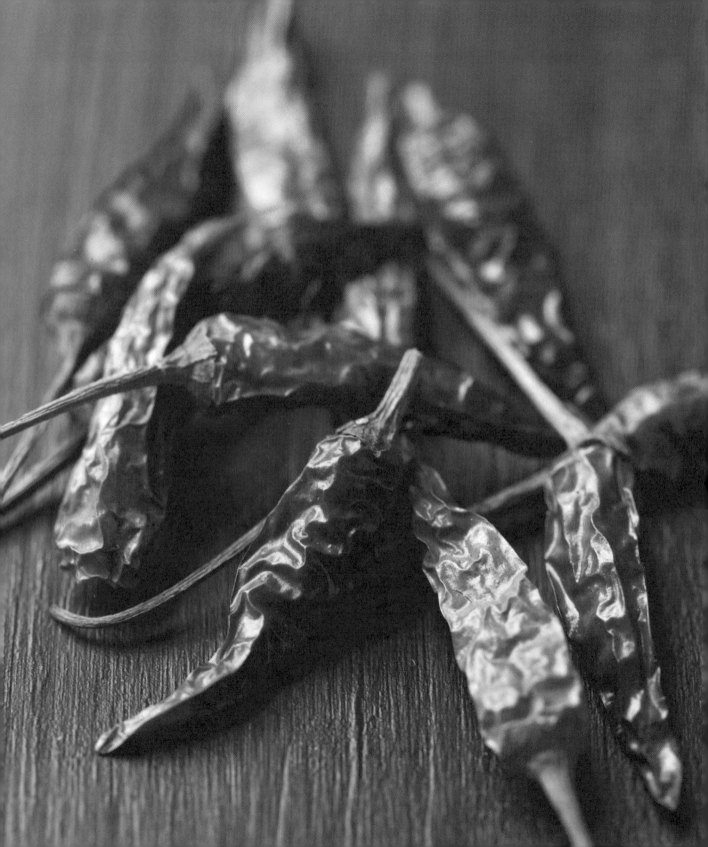

Walnut Chili Pâté Pre-soak

This pâté comes from Green Taco Fusion Fridays in the days of the Gorilla Food take-away window.

⅞ cup (210 mL) sunflower seeds
⅔ cup (160 mL) walnuts
1 celery stalks, chopped
¼ zucchini, chopped
⅜ cup (90 mL) chopped cilantro
¼ cup (60 mL) chopped parsley

1 tbsp lemon juice
⅜ tsp salt
¼ tsp ground cayenne
⅜ tsp chili powder
⅛ tsp ground cumin
⅛ tsp ground coriander

1. In a bowl, soak seeds and walnuts for 6–8 hours or overnight and rinse well before using.

2. In a food processor with an s-blade, process seeds and walnuts until coarse but sticky. Place in a bowl.

3. In a food processor with an s-blade, process rest of ingredients until soupy, then add to seed and nut mix and combine until well-mixed.

Makes 1¾ cups (415 mL).

Pre-soak

Herb & Cashew Cream Cheez

This one is great as a dip for every vegetable that I can think of!

1 cup (250 mL) cashews
¼ medium zucchini, chopped
1½ tbsp Hemp Seed Basil Pesto (p. 80)

¾ cup (185 mL) chopped cilantro
¼ tsp salt
2 tbsp orange juice

1. In a bowl, soak cashews for 2–5 hours and rinse well before using.

2. In a food processor with an s-blade, process all ingredients until creamy.

Makes 1½ cups (375 mL).

 Pre-soak

Sunny Garlic Rawcotta

I can't help but eat a few scoops of this whenever I make a lasagna.

3¼ cups (810 mL) sunflower seeds
2 garlic cloves

⅞ tsp salt
⅞ cup (310 mL) olive oil

1. In a bowl, soak seeds for ½–4 hours and rinse well before using.

2. In a food processor with an s-blade, mince garlic.

3. Add seeds, salt, and olive oil. Process until seeds are sticky but still a little chunky.

Makes 4 cups (1 L) or enough for 1 lasagna recipe (see p. 146).

Blueberry Cream Cheez

So creamy! So fresh! A sweet filling for a berry crêpe or as a spread for the Cinnamon Apple Flax Crackers (p. 43). This always takes me back to the cream cheese at the bagel shop I frequented growing up.

⅔ cup (160 mL) cashews
4–5 dates, pitted

1 tbsp coconut oil
1¼ cups (310 mL) blueberries

1. In a bowl, soak cashews for 2–4 hours and rinse well before using.

2. In a food processor with an s-blade, process all ingredients until whipped into a cream.

Makes 1½ cups (375 mL).

Dilly Brazilly Cream Pre-soak

Dill has such a unique, fresh flavor. This is a great spread for a sandwich, nori roll, or crêpe.

1 cup (250 mL) Brazil nuts
¾–1 medium zucchini, chopped
6 sprigs fresh dill

½ sweet bell pepper
⅜ tsp salt
¼ cup lemon juice

1. In a bowl, soak Brazil nuts for 2 hours or overnight.

2. In a food processor with an s-blade, process all ingredients until smooth.

Makes 1¾–2 cups (415–500 mL).

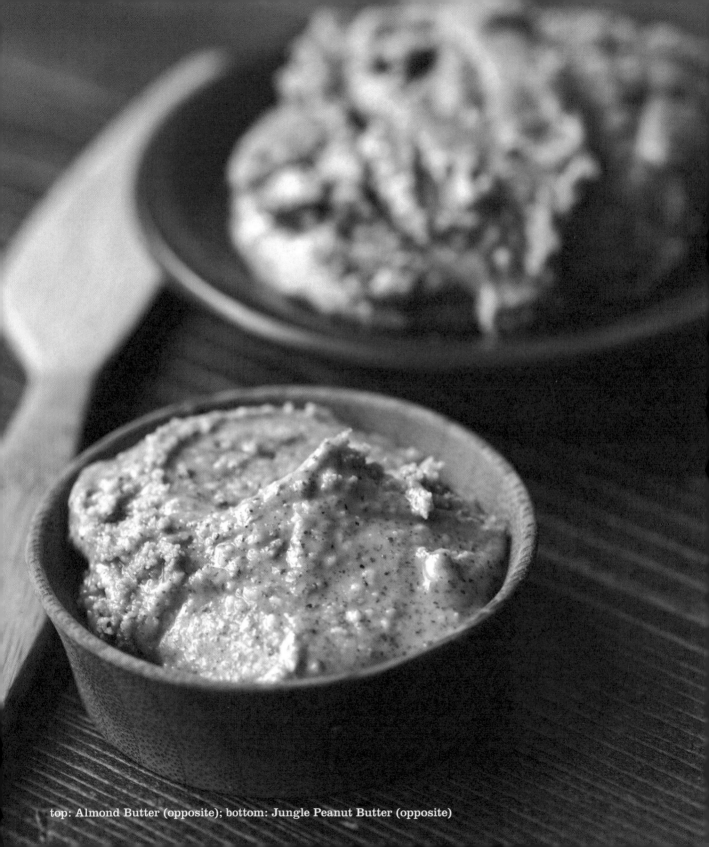

top: Almond Butter (opposite); bottom: Jungle Peanut Butter (opposite)

Almond Butter

Seed and nut butters are great to have pre-prepared to save time. They're nutritious and add a creaminess to sauces, dressings, and dips.

2 cups (500 mL) almonds

1. In a food processor with an s-blade, process almonds to a creamy, smooth consistency. If they heat up before finishing, place in the fridge to cool and then continue to process again until creamy.

Makes 1¾–2 cups (415–500 mL).

Jungle Peanut Butter

Jungle peanuts are an heirloom variety that come from Ecuador. They are a good source of protein and healthy oils.

2 cups (500 mL) jungle peanuts

1. In a food processor with an s-blade, process peanuts to a creamy, butter consistency. If they heat up before finishing, place in the fridge to cool and then continue to process again until creamy.

Makes 1¾–2 cups (415–500 mL).

Hemp Seed Nogurt

A super nourishing sauce with a little tartness, this is a great replacement for dairy yogurt or sour cream. Serve with something sweet or as a contrast to a spicy, savory dish.

4 tbsp hemp seeds
½ cup (125 mL) water
1 date, pitted
2 tbsp lemon juice

1. In a blender, purée all ingredients until well-blended and creamy.

Makes ¾–1 cup (185–250 mL).

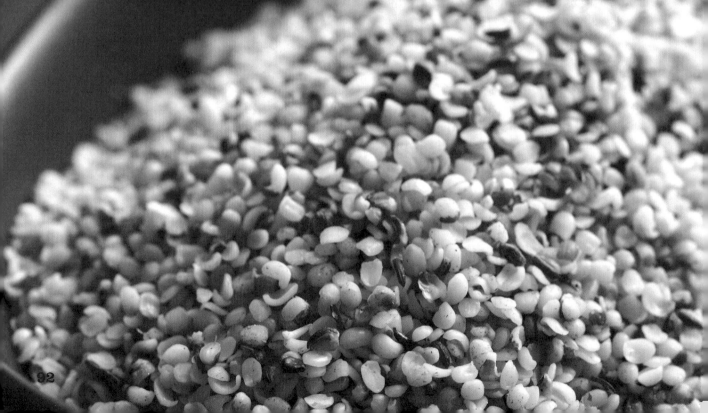

Vanilla Cashew Cream Pre-soak

Use this cream on a fruit salad, as a frosting, or anywhere else you'd want to find sweet creamy stuff!

2 cups (500 mL) cashews
9 dates, pitted
½ cup (125 mL) water
1½ tsp vanilla powder

1. In a bowl, soak cashews for 2–6 hours and rinse well before using.

2. In a food processor with an s-blade, process cashews with rest of ingredients until very smooth and creamy.

Makes 2¼ cups (530 mL).

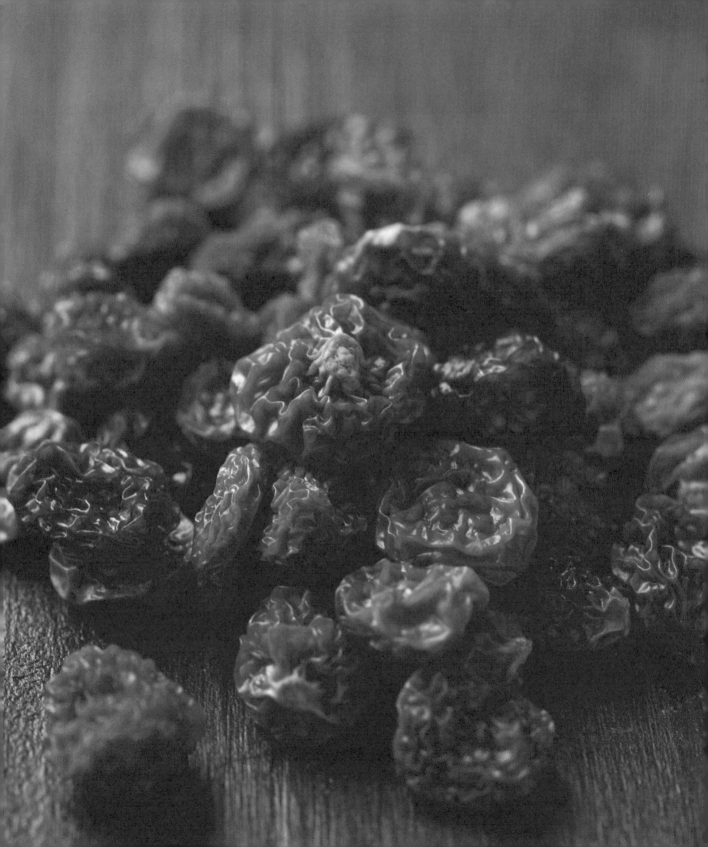

Fruit Compote Syrups Pre-soak

These can be used to replace syrup on Pancakes (p. 30) or to decorate any dessert such as pie or cheezcake. No sugar needed! Use 2–3 tbsp less water to make them thicker (like a jam). They're good for the winter when fruit choices are not as bountiful as in the summer. They're also great in squeeze bottles to use for color accenting or edible decorative designs.

Choose any of the following flavor combinations:
½ cup (125 mL) dried goji berries + 1 cup (250 mL) water
½ cup (125 mL) dried figs + 1 cup (250 mL) water
½ cup (125 mL) dried mangos + 2 cups (500 mL) water
6 dates, pitted + 1 cup (250 mL) water
½ cup (125 mL) dried apricots + 1 cup (250 mL) water
½ cup (125 mL) dried goldenberries + ½ cup (125 mL) water
½ cup (125 mL) dried pineapple + 1½ cup (375 mL) water
½ cup (125 mL) chopped fresh strawberries + 1 cup (250 mL) water
½ cup (125 mL) fresh blueberries + 1 cup (250 mL) water

1. In separate bowls, soak fruits in specified quantities of water for 30–60 minutes.

2. In blender, purée each bowl of fruit and water separately until liquefied.

Each makes between ¾–1½ cups (185–375 mL).

Avocado Frosting

If you're ever in need of rich vegan chocolate frosting, here is your go-to recipe! Super delish and creamy.

4 dates, pitted
2 tbsp coconut oil
¼ tsp vanilla powder

1½ avocados
½ cup (125 mL) cacao powder

1. In a food processor with an s-blade, process dates and coconut oil to a smooth toffee-like consistency.

2. Add all other ingredients and process until creamy and smooth.

Makes 1 cup (250 mL).

Goji Coconut Frosting

This frosting is my favorite on the Cinnamon Almond Crunch Cookies (p. 189). Its unique color is beautiful and eye-catching.

1⅔ cup (410 mL) coconut flakes
3 dates, pitted

¼ cup (60 mL) goji berries
3 tbsp coconut oil

1. In a food processor with an s-blade, process all ingredients except coconut oil to a smooth cream.

2. Add oil and process until smooth.

Makes 1¾–2 cups (415–500 mL).

Spiced Cashew Cream Frosting

This is not only the frosting for the Carrot Cake (p. 216), but it can also be used over fruit salads, cookies, pancakes, or any other desserts! The recipe makes exactly enough for one Carrot Cake.

2 cups (500 mL) cashews	⅛ tsp ground nutmeg
9 dates, pitted	¼ tsp ground cinnamon
½ cup (125 mL) water	⅛ tsp ground cloves

1. Soak cashews for 2–6 hours and rinse well before using.

2. In a food processor with an s-blade, process cashews with the dates, water, and spices until super smooth and creamy.

Makes 2¼ cups (530 mL).

Walnut Cream Frosting

We use this fruit-sweetened frosting on the Orange Walnut Spice cookies (p. 194).

1 cup (250 mL) walnuts	⅜ tsp ground cinnamon
3 tbsp orange juice	5 dates, pitted

1. In a bowl, soak walnuts for 2 hours and rinse well before using.

2. In a food processor with an s-blade, blend all ingredients until creamy and smooth.

Makes 1¼ cups (310 mL).

Fresh Cherry Avocado Mousse

As my friend farmer Fred says, "I pray I'll see another cherry season!" Get 'em while you can, as the season comes and goes quickly! Serve in a bowl as a cobbler filling, pour into a pie crust, or use for layering in a parfait glass.

1½ cups (375 mL) cherries, pitted
¼ tsp orange zest
⅜ cup (90 mL) orange juice
½-in (1-cm) piece ginger
1–1½ avocados

1. In a food processor with an s-blade, blend all ingredients until creamy and smooth.

Makes 2 cups (500 mL).

Dark Cherry Avocado Mousse

This is great on its own or as a layer in parfait glasses.

⅓–½ cup (80–125 mL) dried cherries
1 pinch dried orange zest powder
2–3 dates, pitted
1 tbsp orange juice
¾ tsp grated ginger
1–1½ avocados

1. In a bowl, soak cherries in ½ cup (125 mL) water for 1–2 hours. Reserve soaking water.

2. In a food processor with an s-blade, process the soaked cherries and soaking water into a paste.

3. Add all other ingredients and blend until smooth and creamy.

Makes 1½ cups (375 mL).

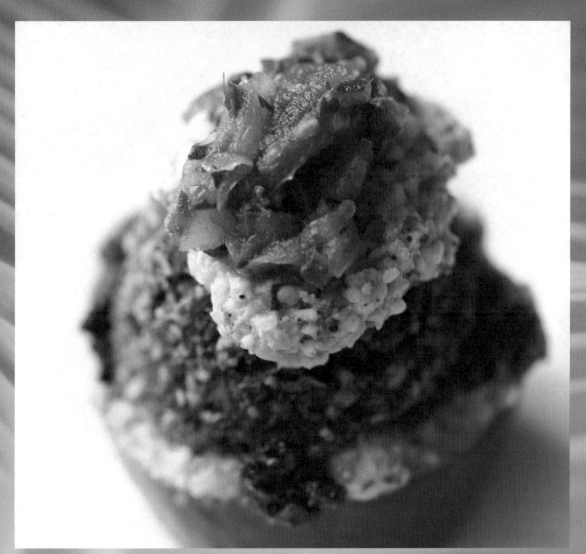

Appetizers & Snacks

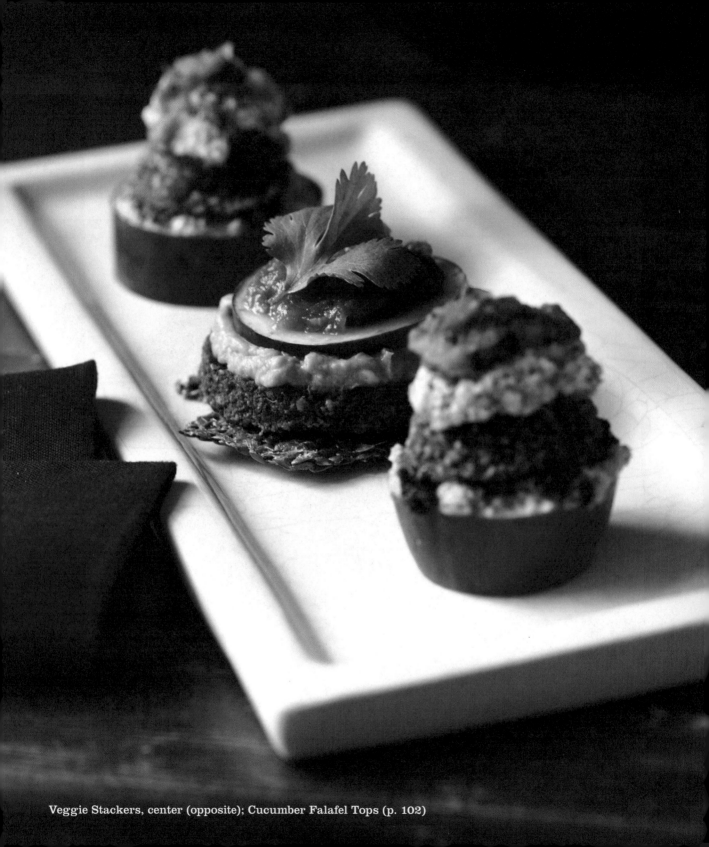

Veggie Stackers, center (opposite); Cucumber Falafel Tops (p. 102)

Veggie Stackers

A great item for finger food, as a snack, or even a light meal.

6 Tomato Herb Flax Crackers (p. 51) or other cracker
  of your choice
6 Veggie Burger Patties (p. 158)
¾ cup (185 mL) Guacamole (p. 78)
6 cucumber slices
¾–1 cup (185–250 mL) Jah Makin Curry Sauce (p. 164) or
  Fresh Ketchup (p. 83)

1. Break up crackers so they are just a bit bigger than burger patties.

2. Center a burger on top of each cracker and dollop with guacamole.

3. Set cucumber slices on top of guacamole.

4. Dollop sauce or ketchup on top of cucumber slices.

Makes 6 servings.

Cucumber Falafel Tops

These make great finger food for parties or as a snack.

6 (¾-in ([2-cm]) thick cucumber slices
2 tbsp–¼ cup (60 mL) Zucchini Hummus (p. 75)
2 tbsp–¼ cup (60 mL) Monkey Tapenade (p. 77)
6 Falafel Balls (p. 169)
6 tsp Tahini Drizzle (p. 69)
6 tsp Salsa (p. 79)

1. With a spoon, scoop seeds out of each cucumber slice to create a hollowed out center, leaving a "bowl".

2. Dollop 1–2 tsp of Zucchini Hummus into each cucumber slice.

3. Dollop 1–2 tsp of Monkey Tapenade on top.

4. Set a Falafel Ball into hummus and tapenade.

5. Drizzle the falafel ball with tahini.

6. Garnish each with 1 tsp of salsa.

Makes 6 tops.

Sauerkraut

Cultured foods are a good way to give yourself a healthy dose of beneficial bacteria. The enzymes and bacteria in cultured cabbage will enhance life-force and aid in the cleansing and metabolic functions of the body.

3 tsp salt
3 heads green and/or red cabbage, shredded

1. In a large bowl, sprinkle salt over cabbage.

2. Squeeze and knead cabbage repeatedly until it releases its juices; when you push down on it, the cabbage should be submerged in the liquid.

3. Add cabbage and juices to a fermentation crock and place weight stones on top to keep cabbage submerged in liquid. Cover with lid and fill crock with water.

4. Leave to sit at room temperature for 11 days; re-fill crock with water as necessary. Give your growing culture positive energy as often as possible.

Makes approx. 15 cups (3¾L).

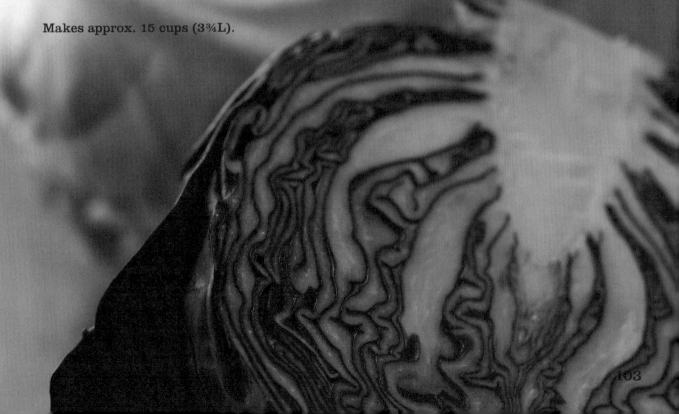

Circa Loco Tops

These delicious triangles will drive you crazy! They were a last-minute creation (along with Coconut Lemon Butter, p. 83) for a catering job, but now I make these on a regular basis because they're so good.

⅓ cup (80 mL) Coconut Lemon Butter (p. 83)
1 piece Curry Squash Bread (p. 36), cut into 4
  or 8 triangles
½ cup (125 mL) Apple Chutney (p. 81)

1. Spread butter onto bread triangles.

2. Top each triangle with approximately 1 tbsp chutney.

Makes 1 serving (4–8 tops).

Olive & Love Veggie Fresh Wraps

These rolls are served at Gorilla Food with Raisin Chutney (p. 81). It's a top pick.

3 collard green leaves
⅜ cup (90 mL) Basic Olive Tapenade (p. 76)
⅜ cup Zucchini Hummus (p. 75)
6 red bell pepper strips (about ½ in [1 cm])
6 cucumber strips (about ½ in [1 cm])
1½ cups (375 mL) sprouts (alfalfa, clover,
  sunflower, etc.)

1. Wash collard leaves and cut each leaf from its thick center stem, leaving 2
   pieces; you will have 6 collard wrappers.

2. Place 1 tbsp of tapenade and 1 tbsp hummus onto each collard leaf.

3. Place a strip of bell pepper and cucumber and ¼ cup (60 mL) sprouts across the
   tapenade and hummus.

4. Roll each leaf up tightly like a cigar.

Makes 6 wraps.

Primo Pesto Wraps

Here is another version of a collard leaf wrap. The Hemp Seed Basil Pesto is rich in healthy fats and primo flavor. This is a quick and convenient way to get more greens into your life.

3 collard green leaves
⅜ cup (90 mL) Hemp Seed Basil Pesto (p. 80)
6 (½-in [1 cm]) tomato strips
6 (½-in [1 cm]) cucumber strips
1½ cups (375 mL) sprouts (alfalfa, clover, sunflower, etc.)
salt, to taste

1. Wash collard leaves and cut each leaf from its thick center stem, leaving 2 pieces; you will have 6 collard wrappers.

2. Place a 1-tbsp dollop of pesto onto each collard leaf.

3. Place a strip of tomato and cucumber and ¼ cup (60 mL) sprouts across the pesto and sprinkle a pinch of salt over top.

4. Roll each leaf up tightly like a cigar.

Makes 6 wraps.

Thai Fresh Wraps

These have remained a go-to dish for me from before I started the restaurant. They are a raw interpretation of some "fresh rolls" that I loved for their tamari-fried tofu and chutney.

3 collard green leaves
½–⅔ cups (125–160 mL) Thai Wrap Pâté (p. 84)
2 cups (500 mL) Sesame Seasoned Coleslaw (p. 122)
½ cup (125 mL) Raisin Chutney (p. 81)

1. Wash collard leaves and cut each leaf from its thick center stem, leaving 2 pieces; you will have 6 collard wrappers.

2. Place 1 tbsp of pâté onto each collard leaf.

3. Place ⅓ cup (80 mL) coleslaw onto pâté.

4. Roll each leaf up tightly like a cigar.

5. Garnish each roll with 1 tbsp chutney.

Makes 6 rolls.

Salt & Vinegar Zucchini Chips

These are great to toss on a salad, or for snacking.

2 medium zucchinis, washed and
 stemmed, sliced lengthwise
1 tbsp olive oil

1 tbsp apple cider vinegar
⅔ tsp salt

1. With a knife or mandoline, or in a food processor with a slicing disc, cut zucchini into half-moon slices. Place in a large bowl.

2. Toss zucchini with oil, vinegar, and salt until combined well.

3. Spread zucchini on a mesh sheet and dehydrate at 108°F (42°C) for about 24 hours or until dried.

Makes 8 servings.

Spicy Zucchini Chips

Zucchini chips were one of the first experiments I made when I got a dehydrator. They're nice to have around as a spicy snack or sprinkled over salad.

2 medium zucchinis, washed and
 stemmed, sliced lengthwise
1 tbsp olive oil

1⅓ tbsp apple cider vinegar
2 tbsp Southern Fire Hot Sauce (p. 67)
½ tsp salt

1. With a knife or mandoline, or in a food processor with a slicing disc, cut zucchini into half-moon slices. Place in a large bowl.

2. Toss zucchini with oil, vinegar, hot sauce and salt until combined well.

3. Spread zucchini on a mesh sheet and dehydrate at 108°F (42°C) for about 24 hours or until dried.

Makes 8 servings.

Super Sister Savory Kale, Cashew & Herb Chips

I was so surprised—but stoked—to have my sister call me up one day to request kale chips. It assured me that the world is getting better and better!

10 packed cups (2½ L) roughly
  chopped and stemmed kale
1½ cups (375 mL) Cashew Alfredo
  Sauce (p. 65)

½ tsp salt
1 tbsp lemon juice

1. In a bowl, toss kale with rest of ingredients until leaves are evenly covered.

2. Spread kale leaves on a mesh sheet and dehydrate at 108°F (42°C) for about 24 hours or until dried.

Makes 6–8 servings.

Cashew & Herb Tomato Kale Chips

I've had many fun spells making kale chips, and this is the result of one of those times. It's so easy to eat big bowls of these when you have them around!

1 cup (250 mL) cashews
1 tsp salt
⅛ tsp ground black pepper
1½ garlic cloves
½ cup (125 mL) water

2 tbsp lemon juice
2½ tsp dried Italian herbs (parsley,
  basil, oregano, rosemary)
10 packed cups (2½ L) roughly
  chopped and stemmed kale

1. In a blender, purée all ingredients except kale until well-blended and creamy.

2. In a bowl, toss kale with puréed ingredients until evenly covered.

3. Spread kale leaves on a mesh sheet and dehydrate at 108°F (42°C) for about 24 hours or until dried.

Makes 6–8 servings.

PW's Savory Kale Chips

Kale, spirulina, and hemp are all concentrated sources of protein, making these an extra great snack for building the body after exercise.

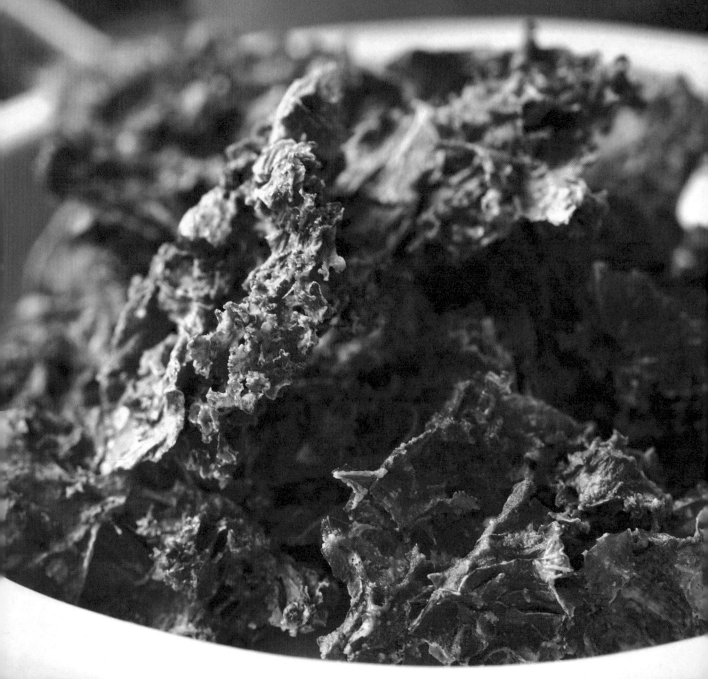

10 packed cups (2½ L) roughly chopped and stemmed kale
½ tsp salt
3 tbsp lemon juice
2 tbsp olive oil
⅜ tsp cayenne chili powder
⅛ tsp ground cumin seed
¼ tsp spirulina
¼ tsp maca powder
½ tsp hemp protein powder

1. In a bowl, toss kale with rest of ingredients until leaves are evenly covered.

2. Spread kale leaves on a mesh sheet and dehydrate at 108°F (42°C) for about 24 hours or until dried.

Makes 6–8 servings.

Samosas

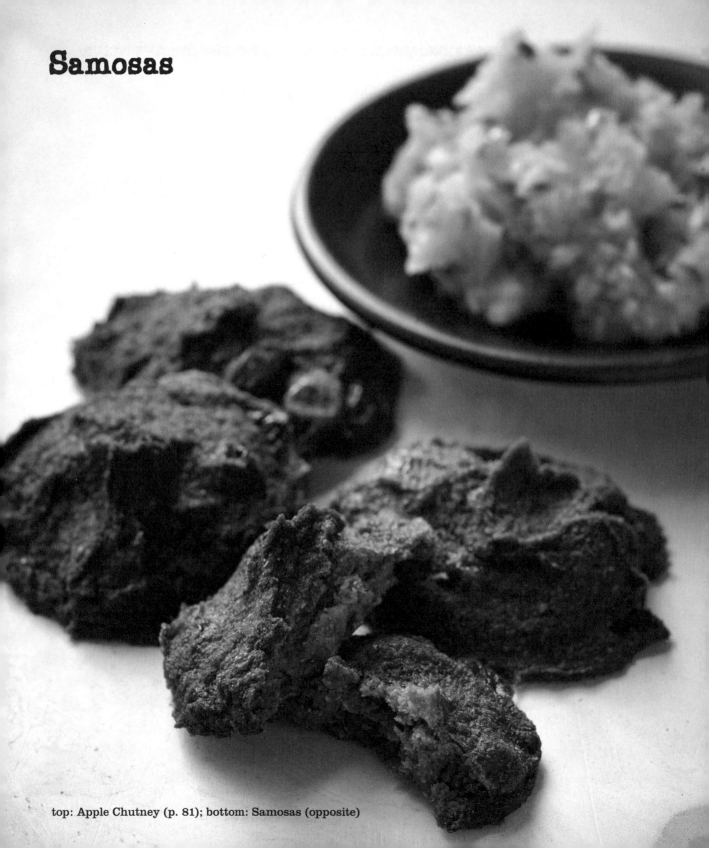

top: Apple Chutney (p. 81); bottom: Samosas (opposite)

Indian food was a staple in my transition to a vegan diet. Even after all these years of raw foods, I still have faint urges to buy a samosa when I'm in the checkout line at Sweet Cherubim, a long-standing vegetarian health food store in Vancouver.

⅓ cup (80 mL) raisins
2⅓ cups (580 mL) chopped cauliflower
1 medium-large zucchini, chopped
⅓ cup (80 mL) chopped parsnips
1–2 collard leaves
⅓ cup (80 mL) chopped sweet bell peppers
⅓ cup (80 mL) chopped cilantro
¾ cup (185 mL) ground flax seeds
2½ tbsp lemon juice

⅛ tsp ground cayenne
1 pinch ground black pepper
¼–½ tsp ground coriander
¼–½ tsp ground turmeric
1 pinch ground cloves
1 tsp ground cumin seeds
1 pinch ground nutmeg
1 tsp salt
⅜ tsp ground cardamom
3 tbsp orange juice

1. In a a bowl, soak raisins for 1–2 hours in ½ cup (125 mL) water.

2. In a food processor with an s-blade, process all ingredients except for raisins. Add to a bowl and stir in raisins by hand.

3. Shape each samosa by hand or with a scoop or mold (about ¼–⅓ cup [60–80 mL] each) onto mesh sheets and dehydrate at 108°F (42°C) for 12–18 hours, until the outside is crusty but the center is still moist.

Makes 18 samosas.

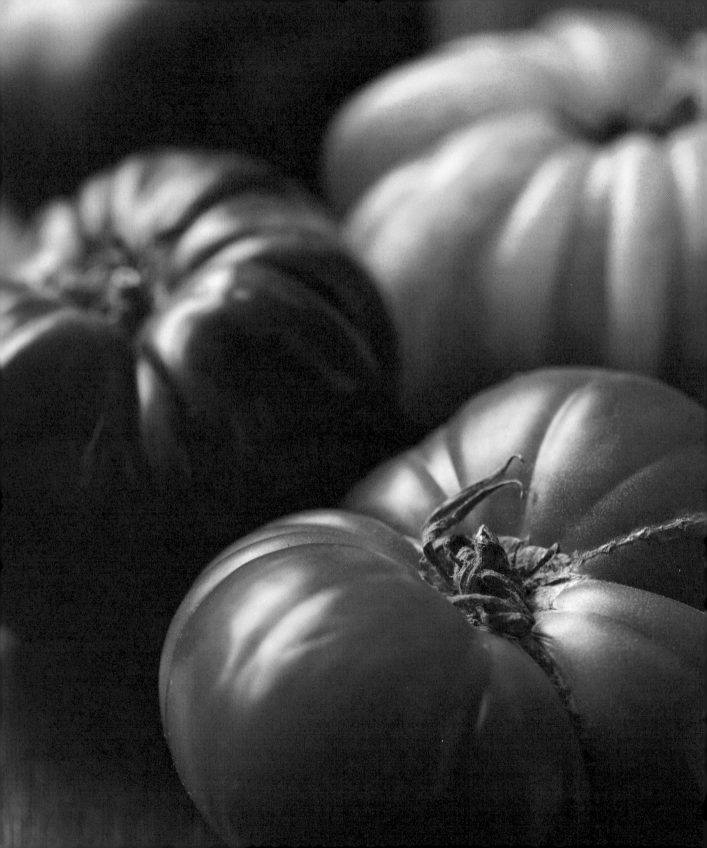

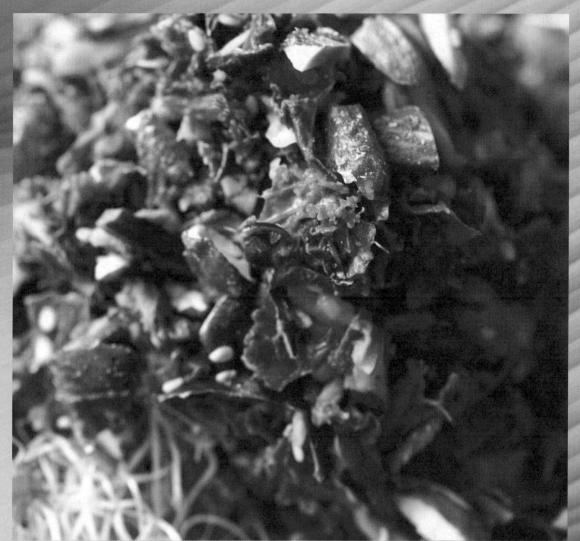

Salads & Soups

Captain Kraut & the Almond Experience

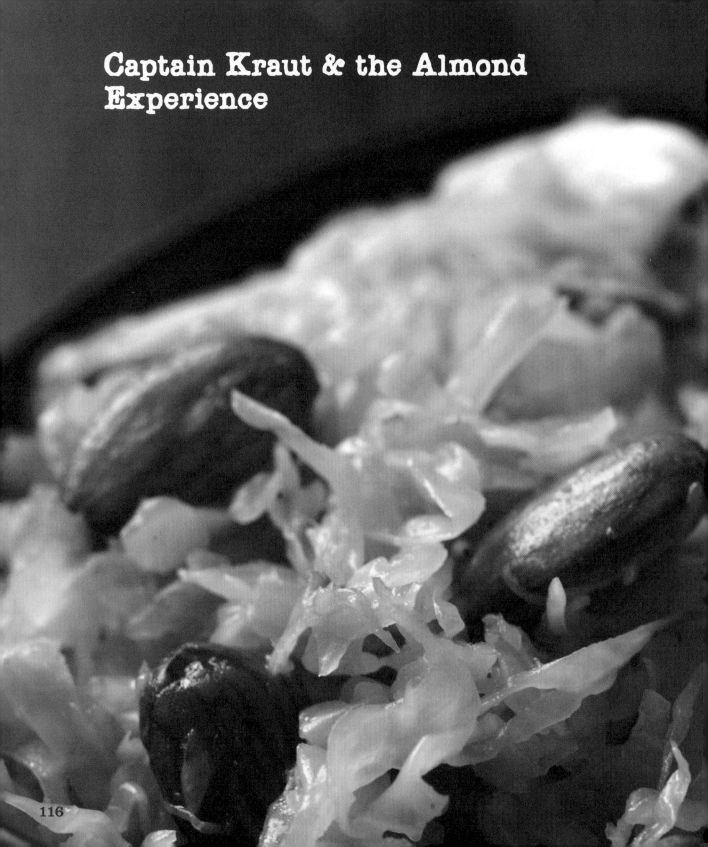

I remember how excited I was when I first bought a fermentation crock. This is a recipe that I made early on, when experimenting with different cultured preparations.

2 cups (500 mL) sauerkraut (make your own or buy an
  unpasteurized organic brand)
3 tbsp orange juice
1–2 tbsp olive oil
⅓ cup (80 mL) sprouted almonds (see p. 131)
2 tbsp sesame seeds

1. Toss all ingredients together in a bowl.

Makes 1–2 servings.

Carrot & Daikon Hemp Seed Toss

A simple salted veggie toss that is a colorful and nutritious element in a maki (nori) roll (p. 171) or any other dish.

2 carrots, shredded
1 (3–4-in [8–10-cm]) long daikon, shredded

3 tbsp hemp seeds
2–3 tsp sesame oil
¾ tsp salt

1. Toss all ingredients together in a bowl.

Makes 1–2 servings.

East Coast West Coast Salad

This one is inspired by a salad I used to enjoy at Radha in Vancouver. Salty East Coast seaweed meets fresh West Coast produce.

1 apple, cored
1 celery stalk
½ cup (125 mL) chopped fennel
¼–⅓ cup (60–80 mL) chopped sunchokes
⅓ cup (80 mL) chopped daikon
¼–½ cup (60–125 mL) chopped (½-in [1-cm]) dulse
⅛ tsp salt
1 tbsp apple cider vinegar
1–2 cups (250–500 mL) Basic Greens Mix (p. 120)

1. With a knife or mandoline or in a food processor with a slicing disc, chop apple, celery, fennel, sunchokes, and daikon.

2. In a large bowl, toss together with dulse, salt, and vinegar.

3. On a plate, lay a bed of greens and then top with apple and dulse mix.

Makes 1–2 servings.

Basic Greens Mix

The contents of this salad can vary throughout the year, depending on what is in season. Mix and match for different tastes and textures and enjoy with any of the dressings, sauces, or goos in this book. Add sprouts! Add olives! Add assorted veggies! Wrap your greens in a nori sheet or a crêpe, or serve them on crackers. Leafy greens are some of the most important and nutritious foods to eat—so eat lots!

2–4 cups (½–1 L) tender leaves (kale, lettuce, chard, spinach, watercress, sprouts, herbs, flowers, etc.)

1. Chop, tear, and combine any assortment of edible greens.

Makes 1–2 servings.

Carrot, Arame, Lime & Pine Nut Salad

 Pre-soak

Mmm-mm, so nourishing! When I created this, I was inspired by a seaweed salad that a friend brought to a dinner party once. It's totally different, yet it still satiates my desire for that salad. Arame is a kind of seaweed often used in Japanese cuisine; you can find it in Asian markets.

1 cup (250 mL) dry arame
3 tbsp lime juice
½ tsp salt
2 cups (500 mL) shredded carrots
½ cup (125 mL) sliced celery
⅜ cup (90 mL) pine nuts
2 tbsp sesame oil

1. Soak arame in water for about 1 hour. Drain and rinse lightly.

2. Toss all ingredients together in a bowl.

Makes 2–4 servings.

Basic Coleslaw Mix

This is a fresh, hydrating, colorful coleslaw that you can add other seasonal veggies to. You can use this mix in many different recipes or dishes. It always reminds me of the big batches of cabbage I would see beside the giant woks in OB Kitchen in Regina, a favorite Chinese take-out restaurant I went to as a kid.

2 carrots, washed and trimmed
2 cups (500 mL) roughly chopped green cabbage
1¼ cups (310 mL) roughly chopped red cabbage

1. In a food processor with a shredding disc, shred carrots.

2. In a food processor with a slicing disc, slice both cabbages.

3. Toss all ingredients in a large bowl until combined well.

Makes 4–5 cups.

Variation: Sesame Seasoned Coleslaw

To Basic Coleslaw Mix, add:

1 tsp salt
¼ cup (60 mL) sesame seeds
1 tbsp sesame oil

1. Add salt, seeds, and oil to coleslaw and toss all ingredients until combined well.

Jungle Slaw

This is another long-standing favorite at Gorilla Food.

⅔ cup (160 mL) chopped avocado
⅓ cup (80 mL) Raisin Chutney (p. 81)
5 cups (1¼ L) Sesame Seasoned Coleslaw (p. 122)

1. In a large bowl, mash avocado with a fork. Stir in chutney until well-combined.

2. Toss coleslaw and add to avocado and chutney. Mix all by hand until well-combined.

Makes 4 servings.

Gado Marinated Veggies

Any combination of vegetables works well with this simple salt and oil marinade. Use whatever is in season.

1 cup (250 mL) chopped (bite-sized) broccoli
1 cup (250 mL) chopped (bite-sized) cauliflower
1 cup (250 mL) chopped (bite-sized) red bell peppers
1 tbsp sesame oil
¼–½ tsp salt

1. In a mixing bowl, toss all ingredients until combined well.

Makes 3 cups (750 mL).

"Seazer" Salad

I have an old roommate (whom I love) who will not be pleased with the name of this salad, but please—I mean no disrespect to the original!

6–8 cups (1½–2L) coarsely chopped or torn romaine lettuce
½ cup (125 mL) Cashew Alfredo Sauce (p. 65)
½–1 tsp spirulina powder
2 nori sheets, cut into 1-in (2½-cm) squares

1. In a large bowl or on a plate, toss lettuce with cashew sauce.

2. Sprinkle with spirulina powder.

3. Sprinkle nori squares over salad.

Makes 2 servings.

Ryce

Rice was a great dish for me to learn how to replicate because I used to love so many rice-centric cuisines before shifting to a raw food diet.

½–1 cup (125–250 mL) peeled and chopped parsnips
¾–1 cup (185–250 mL) chopped broccoli
1 (6–9-in [15–23-cm]) daikon, peeled and chopped
1½ carrots, peeled and chopped
1 celery stalk, chopped
⅓ medium zucchini, chopped
½ cup (125 mL) sesame seeds
¾ tsp salt
2 tbsp sesame oil

1. Cut all vegetables to a consistent size for food processor (about 1–2-in [2½–5-cm] pieces).

2. In a food processor with an s-blade, pulse-process all veggies, seeds, salt, and oil to an approximately rice-sized consistency.

Makes 4 servings.

Grainless Tabouli

A fresh and tasty take on a classic Middle Eastern salad.

1⅓ cups (315 mL) chopped tomatoes
⅔ cup (160 mL) chopped cucumber
½ cup (125 mL) packed parsley, minced
1½ tbsp lemon juice
⅜ tsp salt
1½ tbsp olive oil

1. In a large bowl, combine tomatoes, cucumber, and parsley.

2. Add lemon juice, salt, and olive oil and mix until all ingredients are combined well.

Makes 2½ cups (625 mL).

 Pre-soak

Sprouted Quinoa Tabouli

This is a live alternative to the cooked bulgur wheat in traditional tabouli.

½ cup (125 mL) quinoa
1 cup (250 mL) Grainless Tabouli (above)
¼ tsp salt

1. In a large bowl, soak quinoa overnight or for at least 4–6 hours and rinse with fresh water in a colander. Leave to sprout tails over the next several hours to 2 days, rinsing every 8 hours.

2. Toss sprouted quinoa with tabouli and salt.

Makes 1–2 servings.

Sprouted Quinoa, Tomato & Olive Medley

Serve on a bed of Basic Greens (p. 120) with a scoop of Zucchini Hummus (p. 75).

1 cup (250 mL) quinoa
¼ cup (60 mL) sun-dried tomatoes
¼ cup (60 mL) chopped celery
⅜ cup (90 mL) pitted sun-dried black olives
¼ tsp salt
2 tbsp lime juice

1. In a large bowl, soak quinoa for about 4 hours and rinse well. Leave to sprout tails over the next several hours to 2 days, rinsing every 8 hours.

2. Soak sun-dried tomatoes in water for about 2 hours, until softened.

3. Dice tomatoes.

4. Julienne olives.

5. In a large bowl, toss all ingredients together until combined well.

Makes 1–2 servings.

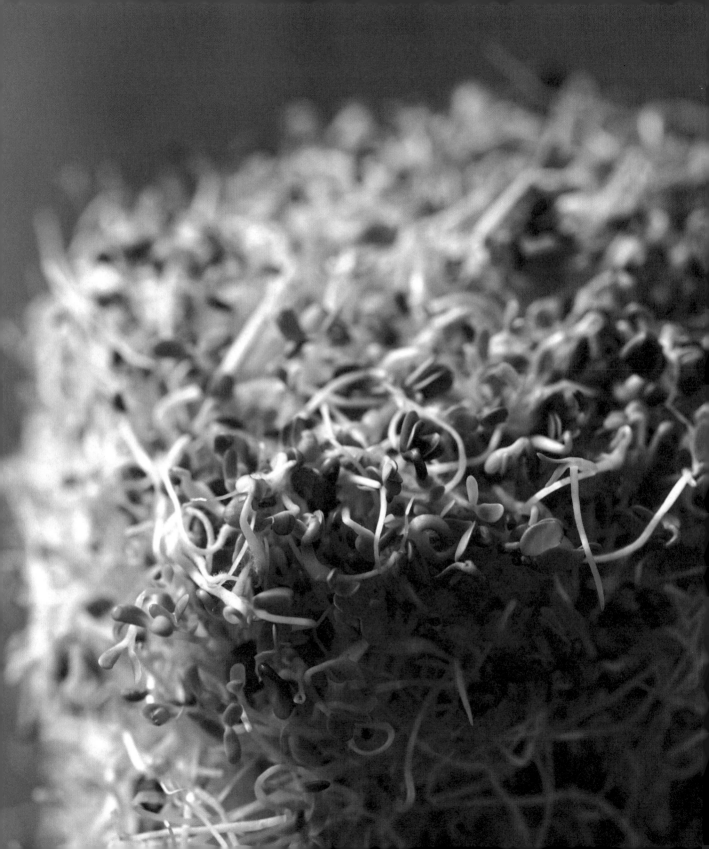

Sprouts

This is the basic way to make most sprouts.

1 tbsp—1 cup (15–250 mL) seeds, nuts, or legumes

1. Soak 1 part seeds in 2 parts water for the appropriate amount of time according to each seed (see table below).

2. Drain and rinse well with fresh water.

3. You can sprout in a bowl, jar, colander, or sprouting device. Rinse well every 8–12 hours, until a tail starts to grow from the seed or bean.

Seed or bean:	Hours to soak:	Days to sprout:
Adzuki bean	12–15	3–5
Alfalfa	6–8	3–5
Almond	8–12	1–3
Buckwheat	6–8	1–2
Chickpea (Garbanzo)	6–8	3–5
Clover	6–8	2–3
Fenugreek	12–15	2–3
Lentil (Brown, Green, Red)	8–12	1–3
Mung bean	12	3–5
Quinoa	4–6	1–3
Sesame	6–8	1–2

The Great Gorilla

When I used to make this for myself, everyone kept asking me what I was eating—that's how this super hearty salad came to be on the menu at Gorilla Food. I love to eat it rolled in nori sheets.

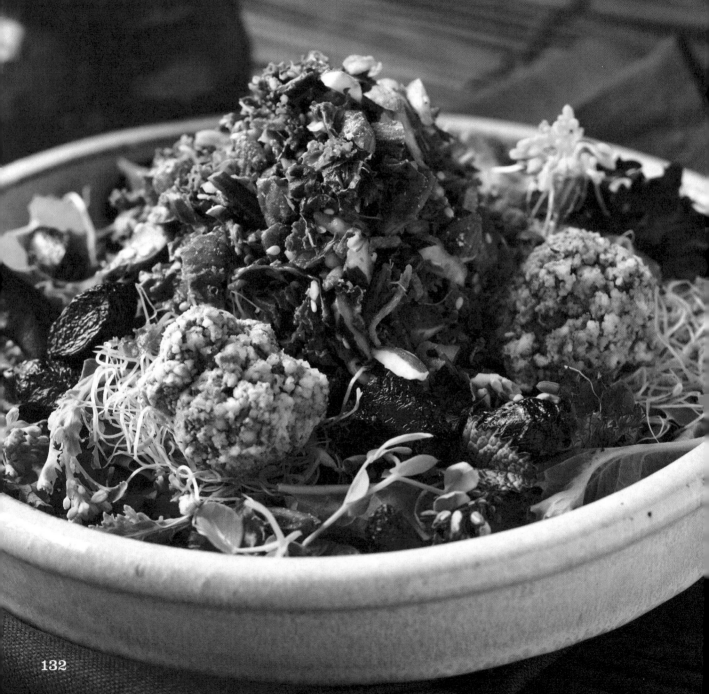

1½ cups (375 mL) Basic Greens Mix (p. 120)
4 tbsp Super-Food Dressing (p. 74)
¾–1 cup (185–250 mL) Jungle Slaw (p. 123)
1½ cups (375 mL) Tossed and Tenderized Deep Greens (p. 134)
½–1 cup (125–250 mL) sprouts (alfalfa, clover, sunflower, etc.)
4 tbsp Thai Wrap Pâté (p. 84)
8–12 pitted sun-dried black olives
3–4 tbsp chopped Chili Almonds (p. 56)

1. On a plate, place a bed of basic greens and drizzle dressing over top.

2. In a bowl, toss together coleslaw and deep greens and layer on top of basic greens.

3. Add sprouts, pâté, and olives over top.

4. Sprinkle with almonds.

Makes 1–2 servings.

Tossed & Tenderized Deep Greens

A core of the Gorilla Food diet! This recipe provides you with a wide variety of greens, along with their minerals and chlorophyll. Anything that's in season can be used in this salad. It is delicious as is, with a dressing, or as an added element in any number of dishes.

3 bunches washed and stemmed dark
leafy greens
  (kale, chard, beet greens, spinach,
  collard, etc.)
½–1 tsp salt

2–3 tbsp lemon juice
1 medium zucchini
1 red bell pepper
2–3 tbsp minced onions

1. With a knife, cut greens into small ribbons.

2. In a large bowl, combine greens with salt and lemon juice.

3. Hand squeeze greens to tenderize until they take on a wilted or steamed-like quality.

4. Medium-dice zucchini and bell pepper into ½-in (1-cm) niblets and toss with onions and greens.

Makes 3–6 cups (¾–1½ L).

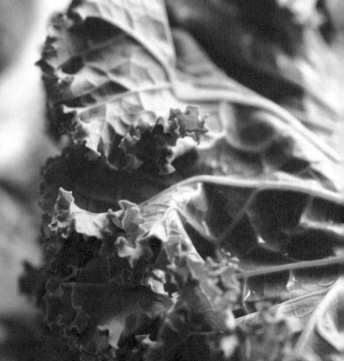

Guacamole & Greens

We use this as a layer in sandwiches at the restaurant. It's also great as a salad on its own. You can serve it with crackers (pp. 41-52) or cut nori sheets.

2½ cups (625 mL) Tossed and Tenderized Deep Greens (p. 134)
½ cup (125 mL) Guacamole (p. 78)

1. In a bowl, toss ingredients until combined well.

Makes 2–3 cups (500–750 mL).

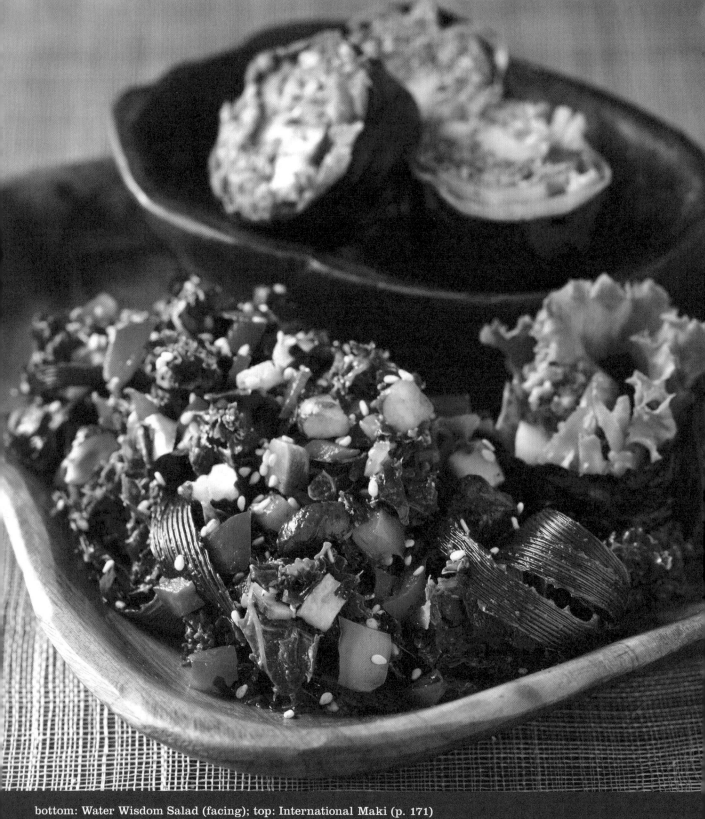

bottom: Water Wisdom Salad (facing); top: International Maki (p. 171)

Water Wisdom Salad

Soaking the salty seaweed in sweet carrot juice was a tip I picked up from a seaweed harvester once. That was a great gift! This has been a favorite for many people over the years.

1–1½ apples
1–1½ carrots
¼-in (½-cm) piece ginger
¾ cup (185 mL) cut or torn (1-in [1½-cm] pieces)
  mixed seaweeds (nori, wakame, dulse, sea palm, etc.)
⅓ cup (80 mL) coarsely chopped hazelnuts
¼ cup (60 mL) sesame seeds
2 tbsp sesame oil
4 cups (1 L) Tossed and Tenderized Deep Greens (p. 134)

1. Press apples, carrots, and ginger through a juicer and pour juice into a large bowl.

2. Soak seaweed, hazelnuts, and sesame seeds in juice for at least 1 hour. Seaweed will double in size after being soaked.

3. Stir in sesame oil.

4. Add greens and toss until combined well.

Makes 2–4 servings.

Dreamy Cream Avocado Carrot & Basil Soup

One of the first raw soups I ever made was carrot and avocado soup, which is very refreshing on a hot summer day. Top each bowl with a large pinch of Carrot & Daikon Hemp Seed Toss (p. 118). You can serve this with Veggie Flax Bread (p. 35) and a dollop of Zucchini Hummus (p. 75) on the side.

3 carrots, chopped
¾–1 cup (185–250 mL) packed fresh basil
¼ cup (60 mL) walnuts
2 tbsp hemp seeds
1 tbsp olive oil
2 tsp flax oil
¼–½ cup (60–125 mL) chopped avocado
½ tsp salt
1 tbsp lemon juice
3 cups (750 mL) water

1. In a blender, process all ingredients until smooth.

Makes 2–4 servings.

Chili Verde Soup

I love how clean this soup tastes, and you can use any types of greens to mix it up. It's a good warming soup with spices for the winter.

3 medium kale leaves
5 medium lettuce leaves
1 celery stalk
1 tbsp lemon juice
⅛ tsp ground cayenne
¼ tsp ground cumin
2 tbsp chopped mango
¼ tsp salt
1 cup (250 mL) water

1. In a blender, process all ingredients until smooth.

Makes 1–2 servings.

Green Garden Soup

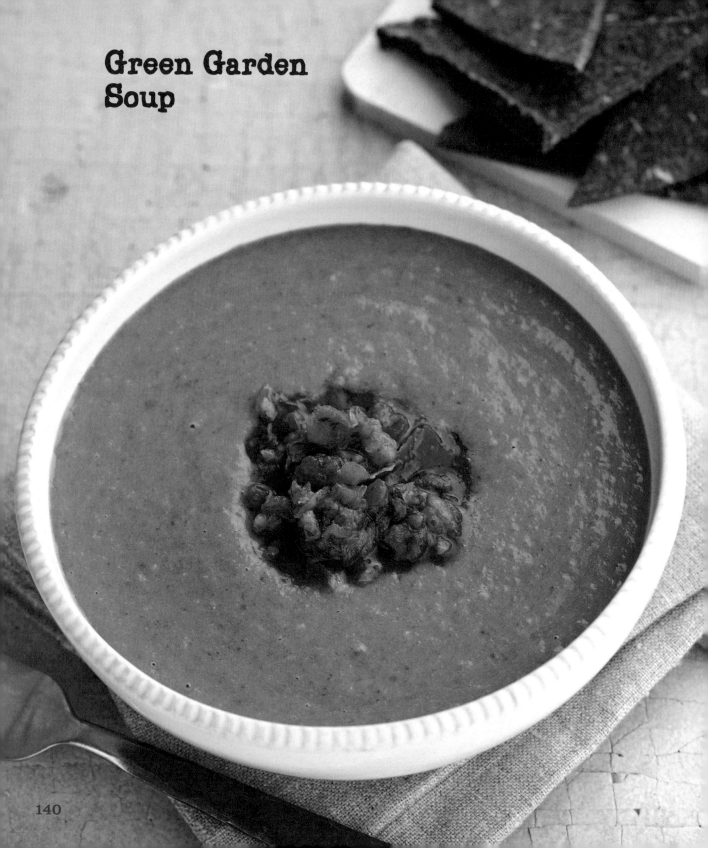

We have an amazing fairy godmother at Gorilla Food who likes to drink her food. This is one of the flavors that has become a standard in her alkalizing diet. You can use tomatoes with fresh herbs instead of the tomato sauce if you don't have any prepared.

2 large handfuls mixed greens (kale, lettuces, chard,
  collards, spinach, etc.)
½ cup (125 mL) Ital Herb Tomato Sauce (p. 66)
2–3 tbsp chopped avocado
¼ tsp salt
1 cup (250 mL) water
½ cup (125 mL) Salsa (p. 79)

1. In a blender, process all ingredients (except salsa) until smooth.

2. Serve in a bowl with salsa in the center for flavor, color, and texture.

Makes 1–2 servings.

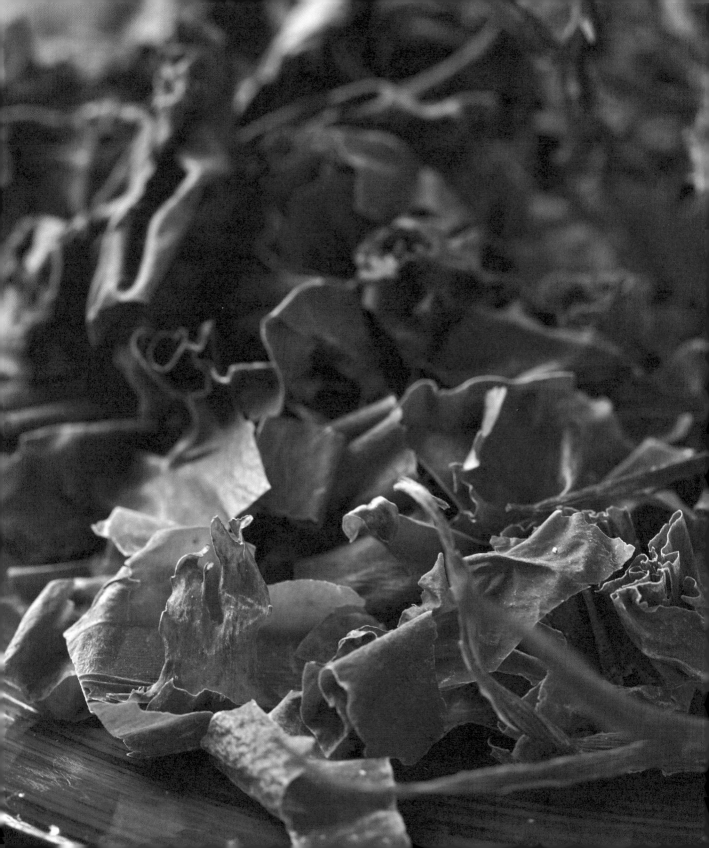

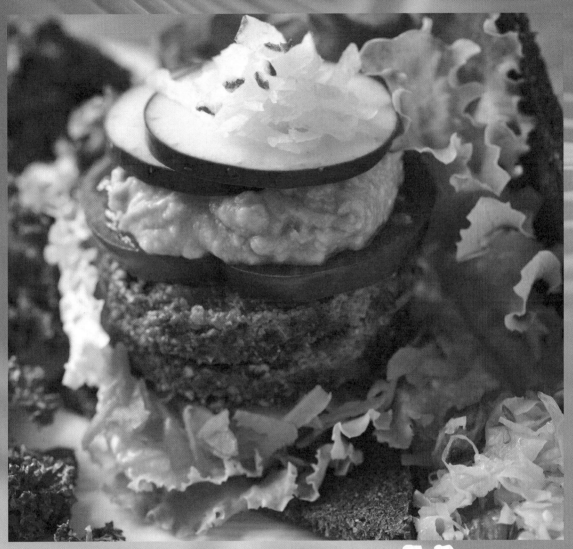

Mains

Cashew Alfredo Zucchini Linguini

Whenever I spin zucchini into "New"dles," I think back to my first restaurant job at Casa Italia where I learned how to toss fettuccini noodles in a pan. Same thing here, only better!

3–4 zucchinis, washed and trimmed
1 cup (250 mL) Cashew Alfredo Sauce (p. 65)

1. Center each zucchini in a Spirooli slicer and spin into "New"dles.

2. Chop "New"dles to shorten the length.

3. In a large bowl, toss the "New"dles well by hand with the sauce.

Makes 2–4 servings.

Kunda Linguini Rising

Raise up your life-force!

2–3 medium zucchinis, washed and trimmed
⅓ cup (80 mL) Hemp Seed Basil Pesto (p. 80)
¾–1 cup (185–250 mL) Ital Tomato Herb Sauce (p. 66)
1 cup (250 mL) Tossed and Tenderized Deep Greens (p. 134)
¾ cup (185 mL) Walnut Cheez Crumble (p. 71)
2–3 tbsp Basic Olive Tapenade (p. 76)

1. Center each zucchini in a Spirooli slicer and spin into "New"dles.

2. Chop "New"dles to shorten the length.

3. In a large bowl, toss "New"dles with pesto.

4. Top with tomato sauce, then add greens.

5. Top with Walnut Cheez and garnish with tapenade.

Makes 3 servings.

J Rawk's Xmas Spaghetti

One year, I made this especially for a regular customer, Mr. J. Rawka, when we were closing over the New Year's break. He was worried about what he would eat without us. It's now one of my favorites!

2–3 medium zucchinis, washed and trimmed
2 tbsp lemon juice
⅛ tsp salt
1 pinch ground cayenne
1 tbsp lucuma powder
2 tbsp Hemp Seed Basil Pesto (p. 145)
2 tbsp olive oil
¼ cup (60 mL) pine nuts
½ cup (125 mL) chopped black sun-dried olives

1. Center zucchini in a Spirooli slicer and spin them into "New"dles.

2. Chop "New"dles to shorten the length.

3. In a large bowl, toss "New"dles with remainder of ingredients.

4. Serve mounded on a plate or in a pasta bowl.

Makes 2 servings.

Lasagna-nanda

Bliss lasagna! This is really good fresh or cold, but also when you warm it for 1–3 hours in the dehydrator.

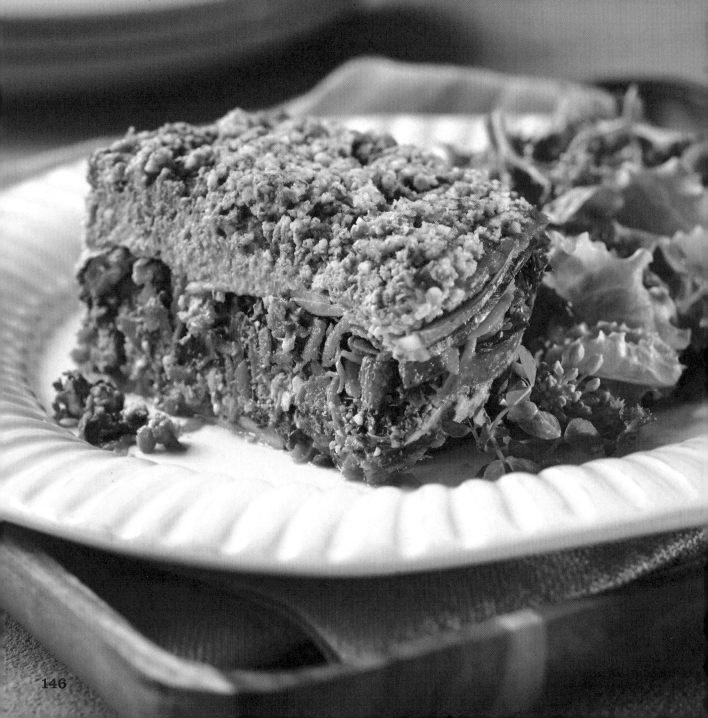

3–4 medium zucchinis, washed and trimmed
4½ cups (1 L + 125 mL) Ital Herb Tomato Sauce (p. 66)
3½–4 cups (830 mL–1 L) shredded carrots
1 cup (250 mL) Hemp Seed Basil Pesto (p. 80)
2⅔ cups (630 mL) Tossed and Tenderized Deep Greens (p. 134)
5 cups (1¼ L) Sunny Garlic Rawcotta (p. 88)
2½ cups (625 mL) Walnut Cheez Crumble (p. 71)

1. With either a knife, mandoline, or food processor with slicing disc, thinly slice zucchinis lengthways into a lasagna-noodle shape.

2. Layer ½ of "New"dles to evenly cover bottom of a 13 x 9-in (33 x 23-cm) lasagna pan, overlapping them slightly.

3. Spread 1½ cups (375 mL) tomato sauce over "New"dles.

4. Cover with ½ of carrots.

5. Drizzle ½ of pesto over carrots and spread evenly.

6. Cover with 1⅓ cups (315 mL) greens.

7. Spread ½ of Rawcotta over greens. Use wet hands to spread and keep from sticking. Press slightly to set layers.

8. Pour and spread another 1½ cups (375 mL) tomato sauce over Rawcotta layer.

9. Add another layer of "New"dles evenly over tomato sauce, overlapping them slightly.

10. Cover "New"dles with another 1⅓ cups (315 mL) greens.

11. Drizzle rest of pesto evenly over top.

12. Spread rest of shredded carrots over top.

13. Spread rest of Rawcotta evenly over top. Use wet hands to spread and keep from sticking. Press down firmly to set layers.

14. Spread rest of tomato sauce over top.

15. Sprinkle Walnut Cheez evenly over top and, with wet hands, firmly press everything down to set layers.

16. Cut into squares.

Makes about 10 servings.

Rawmein "New"dles

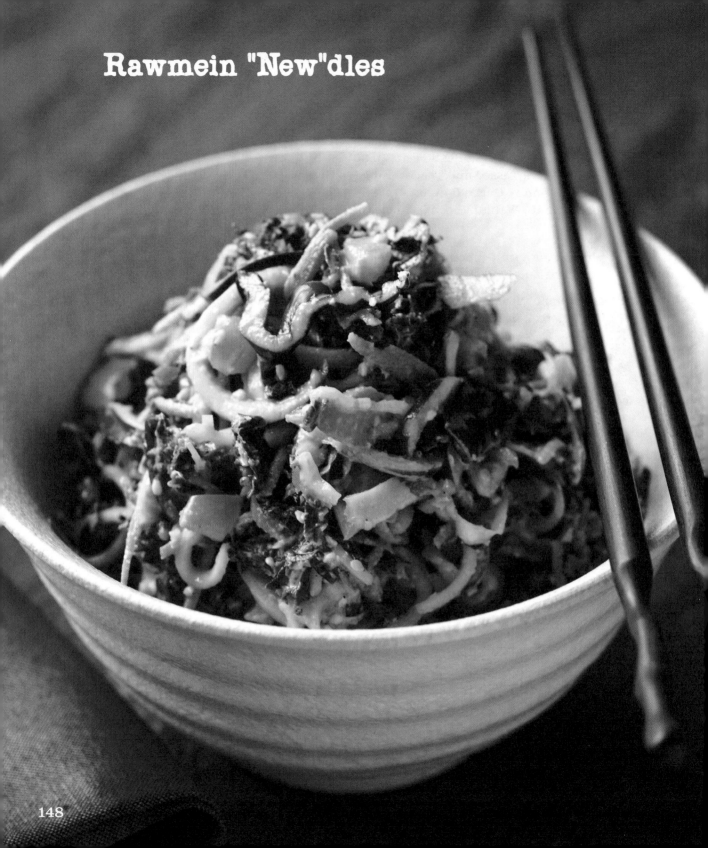

These spicy "New"dles are full of fresh, live enzymes! They can be served in a bowl just as they are or in combination with other foods.

3 medium zucchinis, washed and trimmed
3 cups (750 mL) Sesame Seasoned Coleslaw (p. 122)
3 cups (750 mL) Tossed and Tenderized Deep Greens (p. 134)
1½–1¾ cups (375–415 mL) Nice'n' Spicy Sesame Chili Sauce (p. 67)

1. Center each zucchini in a Spirooli slicer and spin into "New"dles.

2. Chop "New"dles to shorten the length.

3. In a large bowl, toss "New"dles with rest of ingredients to combine well.

Makes 2–4 servings.

Sea Veggie Fettuccini with Macadamia Cream Sauce

The first time I made this was with some friends who brought buckwheat crackers made from a sourdough culture that had been passed on and kept alive for over 100 years. We served it on top of those crackers. Sometimes I make this with arame seaweed instead.

1½ cups (375 mL) sea palm fronds
¾ cup (185 mL) Macadamia Cream Sauce (opposite)
⅓–½ cup (80–125 mL) julienned basil leaves
½–⅔ cup (125–160 mL) chopped cherry tomatoes

1. In a bowl, soak palm fronds in water until softened and plump, about ½–2 hours. Drain and discard water.

2. In a bowl, toss "New"dles in cream sauce.

3. Garnish with basil and tomatoes.

Makes 2 servings.

Sea palm fronds are found on the rugged Pacific coast of North America. You can buy them online and in some specialty or health food stores.

Macadamia Cream Sauce

Pre-soak

Other than some of my favorite people, macadamia nuts are possibly the greatest treasure from the land down under!

1 cup (250 mL) macadamia nuts
½–1 garlic clove
1–2 tbsp lemon juice
½ tsp salt
⅓ cup (80 mL) water

1. In a bowl, soak nuts for 2–4 hours and rinse well before using.

2. In a food processor with an s-blade, process all ingredients until smooth and creamy.

Makes ¾ cup (185 mL).

Sunny Buckwheat Pizza Crusts

This crust is a great base for any pizza. I like to put sauce on and leave it for a couple of hours before eating it so the crust will soften.

4 cups (1 L) buckwheat
3¾ cups (935 mL) sunflower seeds
⅔ cup (160 mL) flax seeds
4 carrots

3½ tbsp dried Italian herbs (parsley, basil, oregano, rosemary)
3½ tsp salt

1. In a bowl, soak buckwheat and sunflower seeds overnight or for at least 6 hours, rinsing well before using.

2. In a blender or coffee grinder, grind flax seeds to a powder.

3. In a food processor with a grater disc, shred carrots.

4. In a food processor with an s-blade, process buckwheat, sunflower seeds, herbs, and salt to a creamy, peanut butter consistency. Pour into a mixing bowl.

5. Add shredded carrots and ground flax seeds and mix thoroughly by hand.

6. Hand-form 4 round (about 13-in [33-cm] diameter) pizza crusts onto ParaFlexx sheets.

7. Mark 6 or 8 slices on each pizza with the back edge of a knife, scoring only halfway deep into the crust.

8. Dehydrate at 108°F (42°C) for 8–12 hours.

9. Flip them over onto mesh sheets and dehydrate at the same temperature for another 24–36 hours or until completely dry.

Makes 4 (13-in [33-cm]) crusts.

Maui Waui Pizza

It used to be all about the Hawaiian, but now it's all about the Maui Waui!

1 Sunny Buckwheat Pizza Crust (p. 152), pre-scored into slices
1–1¼ cup (250–310 mL) Ital Herb Tomato Sauce (p. 66)
4 cups (1 L) Tossed and Tenderized Deep Greens (p. 134)
1 cup (250 mL) Walnut Cheez Crumble (p. 71)
1 cup (250 mL) chopped pineapple

1. Spread tomato sauce evenly over entire pizza crust, to the edges.

2. Distribute greens evenly over top.

3. Sprinkle evenly with Cheez.

4. With wet hands, press toppings down to set.

5. Leave the crust to soften for a few hours before cutting or, with care, cut into pieces.

6. Sprinkle pineapple over top.

Makes 1 (13-in [33-cm]) pizza.

More Rawkin' Olive Pizza

This is a rawkin' pizza! I like to enjoy it with a big scoop of Guacamole (p. 78) on it.

1 Sunny Buckwheat Pizza Crust (p. 152), pre-scored into slices
1 cup (250 mL) Ital Herb Tomato Sauce (p. 66)
4 cups (1 L) Tossed and Tenderized Deep Greens (p. 134)
1 cup (250 mL) Walnut Cheez (p. 71)
⅜–½ cup (90–120 mL) Basic Olive Tapenade (p. 76)
⅜–½ cup crushed Chili Almonds (p. 56)

1. Spread tomato sauce evenly over entire pizza crust, to the edges.

2. Distribute greens evenly over top.

3. Sprinkle evenly with Cheez.

4. With wet hands, press toppings down to set.

5. Leave the crust to soften for a few hours before cutting or, with care, cut into pieces.

6. On each piece, garnish with about 1 tbsp each of tapenade and almonds.

Makes 1 (13-in [33-cm]) pizza.

Peanut Selectah Pizza

This pizza goes great with the Jungle Slaw (p. 123).

1 Sunny Buckwheat Pizza Crust (p. 152), pre-scored into slices
1–1¼ cup (250–310 mL) Ital Herb Tomato Sauce (p. 66)
4 cups (1 L) Tossed and Tenderized Deep Greens (p. 134)
1 cup (250 mL) Walnut Cheez (p. 71)
¾–1 cup (185–250 mL) Gado Selectah Sauce
  (see Oh My Gado Peanut Sauce, p. 68)
2–3 tbsp minced cilantro
1–2 tbsp crushed jungle peanuts

1. Spread tomato sauce evenly over entire pizza crust, to the edges.

2. Distribute greens evenly over top.

3. Sprinkle evenly with Cheez.

4. With wet hands, press toppings down to set.

5. Leave the crust to soften for a few hours before cutting or, with care, cut into pieces.

6. Drizzle Gado Selectah Sauce over top of each piece.

7. Sprinkle with cilantro, then top with peanuts.

Makes 1 (13-in [33-cm]) pizza.

Pesto Pizza

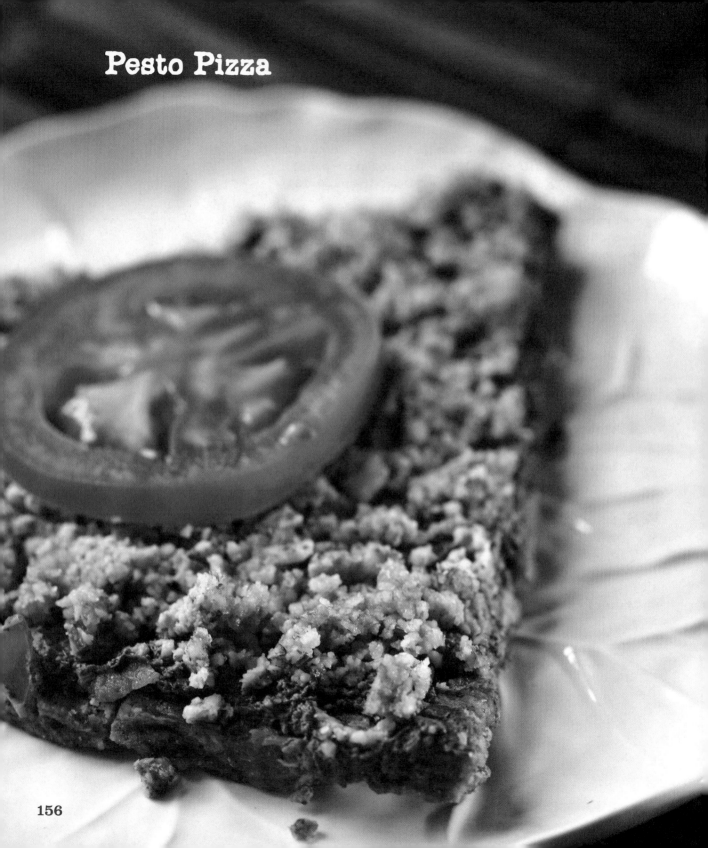

This pizza is a perennial favorite for many customers at Gorilla Food.

1 Sunny Buckwheat Pizza Crust (p. 152), pre-scored into slices
1–1¼ cups (250–310 mL) Ital Herb Tomato Sauce (p. 66)
⅔–¾ cup (160–185 mL) Hemp Seed Basil Pesto (p. 80)
1 cup (250 mL) Walnut Cheez (p. 71)
6 tomato slices

1. Spread tomato sauce evenly over entire pizza crust, to the edges.

2. With a fork, splatter pesto over top, in patches. Then, without mixing it into tomato sauce, spread pesto evenly over top.

3. Sprinkle evenly with Cheez. Press down to set.

4. Carefully following the pre-scored lines, cut into pieces.

5. Top each piece with a tomato slice.

Makes 1 (13-in [33-cm]) pizza.

Variation: Ital Veggie Pizza

Replace Hemp Seed Basil Pesto with 4 cups (1 L) Tossed and Tenderized Deep Greens (p. 134) and omit tomato slices.

Makes 1 (13-in [33-cm]) pizza.

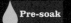 Pre-soak

Veggie Burger Patties

I once had a customer who had many food allergies, but she could eat these patties. They eventually became a popular Thursday special at Gorilla Food's take-away window.

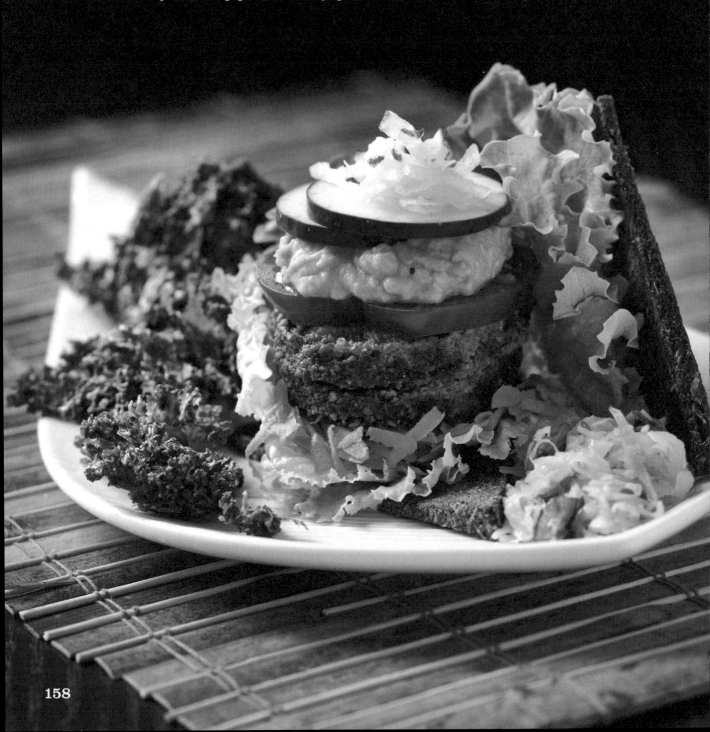

1½ cups (375 mL) walnuts
⅜ cup (90 mL) sunflower seeds
3 tbsp flax seed
3–4 celery stalks
½ red bell pepper, chopped
½ cup (125 mL) chopped onions
2 carrots, chopped
⅔ cup (160 mL) chopped (2-in [5-cm]) tomatoes
¾ tsp salt
1 tbsp hemp protein powder
2 tbsp hemp seeds

1. Soak walnuts and sunflower seeds in water overnight or for about 6 hours and rinse well before using.

2. In a blender or coffee grinder, grind flax seeds into a powder.

3. In a food processor with an s-blade, process celery, bell peppers, onions, carrots, tomatoes, salt, and hemp protein into a soupy purée. Pour into a large bowl.

4. In a food processor, process walnuts and sunflower seeds with just enough of veggie purée to create a paste. Add to rest of veggie purée.

5. Add hemp seeds and ground flax seeds and mix thoroughly by hand.

6. Form mixture into ⅓ cup (80-mL) patties onto mesh sheets.

7. Dehydrate for 18–24 hours at 108°F (42°C) until the outer surfaces are dried but patties are still moist on the inside. Flip them over after about 12 hours to speed up the drying process.

Makes 15 burgers.

Delhi Doubler Burger with Veggie Flax Bun

Some green curry sauce and a bed of dressed veggies make this a nourishing meal.

½ slice Veggie Flax Bread (p. 35), cut in half
2 green lettuce leaves (romaine, butter, etc.)
¼ cup (60 mL) Curry Veggies (p. 165)
2 Veggie Burger Patties (p. 158)
2 tbsp Fresh Ketchup (p. 83)
1 tomato slice
3 tbsp Green Cashew Coconut Curry Sauce (p. 65)
2–3 cucumber slices
1–2 tbsp shredded radish
1–2 tbsp shredded golden beets

1. Set ¼ slice of flax bread onto a plate.

2. Add green lettuce leaf face up, to form a bowl.

3. Place curried veggies inside lettuce leaf.

4. Place burger patty firmly on top. Add 1-tbsp dollop of ketchup.

5. Stack another burger patty on top, then add another 1-tbsp dollop of ketchup and a tomato slice.

6. Dollop curry sauce over tomato and place cucumber slices on top.

7. Top with shredded radish and beets.

8. Place a lettuce leaf over the top or simply lean it against the burger.

9. Top with ¼ slice of flax bread.

Makes 1 burger (1 serving).

GO Veggie Burger with Veggie Flax Bun

I like this one in the lettuce-leaf bun, and if I'm extra hungry, I add the flax bread.

½ slice Veggie Flax Bread (p. 35), cut in half
2 green lettuce leaves (romaine, butter, etc.)
¼ cup (60 mL) shredded carrots
2 Veggie Burger Patties (p. 158)
¼ cup (60 mL) Fresh Ketchup (p. 83)
1 tomato slice
¼ cup (60 mL) Guacamole (p. 78)
2–3 cucumber slices
1–2 tbsp shredded radish
1–2 tbsp shredded golden beets

1. Set ¼ slice of flax bread onto a plate.

2. Add green lettuce leaf face up, to form a bowl.

3. Place shredded carrots inside lettuce leaf.

4. Place burger patty firmly on top. Add 1-tbsp dollop of ketchup.

5. Stack another burger patty on top and add another dollop of ketchup.

6. Add tomato slice and dollop with guacamole. Add layer of cucumber slices.

7. Top with radish and garnish with beets.

8. Place a lettuce leaf over the top or simply lean it against the burger.

9. Top with ¼ slice of flax bread.

Makes 1 burger (1 serving).

Pesto Primo Veggie Burgers with Veggie Flax Bun

This is a nourishing and rich flavorful burger filled with fresh veggies and healthy oils.

½ slice Veggie Flax Bread (p. 35), cut in half
2 green lettuce leaves (romaine, butter, etc.)
¼ cup (60 mL) shredded carrots
3–6 tbsp Hemp Seed Basil Pesto (p. 80)
2 Veggie Burger Patties (p. 158)
1 tomato slice
2 tbsp Fresh Ketchup (p. 83)
2–3 cucumber slices
1–2 tbsp shredded radish
1–2 tbsp shredded golden beets

1. Set ¼ slice of flax bread onto a plate.

2. Add green lettuce leaf face up, to form a bowl.

3. Place shredded carrots in lettuce leaf, then dollop pesto over top.

4. Add burger patty firmly over top then add another dollop of pesto and a tomato slice. Add a dollop of ketchup.

5. Stack another burger patty on top, then add another dollop of pesto. Add cucumber slices.

6. Top with radish and garnish with beets.

7. Place a lettuce leaf over the top or simply lean it against the burger.

8. Top with ¼ slice of flax bread.

Makes 1 burger (1 serving).

Southern Fire Veggie Burger with Veggie Flax Bun

This is the classic—with a little bit of extra spice!

½ slice Veggie Flax Bread (p. 35), cut in half
2 green lettuce leaves (romaine, butter, etc.)
¼ cup (60 mL) shredded carrots
3–4 tbsp Southern Fire Hot Sauce (p. 67)
2 Veggie Burger Patties (p. 158)
¼ cup (60 mL) Salsa (p. 79)
1 tomato slice
¼ cup (60 mL) Guacamole (p. 78)
2–3 cucumber slices
1–2 tbsp shredded radish
1–2 tbsp shredded golden beets

1. Set ¼ slice of flax bread onto a plate.

2. Add green lettuce leaf face up, to form a bowl.

3. Place shredded carrots in lettuce leaf and dress with hot sauce.

4. Place burger patty firmly on top and add dollop of salsa.

5. Stack another burger patty, and add another dollop of salsa.

6. Place tomato slice on top, and add dollop of guacamole. Add cucumber slices.

7. Top with radish and garnish with beets.

8. Place a lettuce leaf over the top or simply lean it against the burger.

9. Top with ¼ slice of flax bread.

Makes 1 burger (1 serving).

Jah Makin Curry Sauce

This recipe was originally created for a catering event as part of the sauce for a Caribbean-style veggie and Ryce dish. It is also good dolloped over the Veggie Stackers (p. 101).

¼ cup (60 mL) chopped pineapple
½-in (1-cm) piece ginger
¾ cup (185 mL) chopped tomatoes
1 pinch ground clove
1 pinch ground coriander
1 cardamom pod

1 pinch ground cumin
2–3 tbsp fresh chopped cilantro
1 pinch ground allspice
½ tsp salt
1 pinch ground cayenne
1 tbsp orange juice

1. In blender, purée all ingredients until smooth.

Makes 1 cup (250 mL).

Curry Veggie Nice Bowl

This is one you can let the seasons dictate by adding peas, beans, bok choy, various sprouts, or whatever other veggies are in season.

2 cups (500 mL) Ryce (p. 126)
3–4 cups (750 mL–1 L) Curry Veggies (p. 165)
½–⅔ cup (125–160 mL) Green Cashew Coconut Curry Dressing (p. 65)
1 cup (250 mL) sprouts (alfalfa, clover, sunflower, etc.)

1. In a bowl, place a mound of Ryce.

2. Surround the Ryce with curry veggies.

3. Dollop dressing over top.

4. Garnish with sprouts.

Makes 2 servings.

Curry Veggies

These marinated veggies can be eaten in a Nice Bowl (p. opposite), as a salad, a sabji (curry), or a filling for a wrap. Try changing up the ingredients seasonally with what is available in the garden or at the farmers' market.

5 cups (1¼ L) Tossed and Tenderized Deep Greens (p. 134)
2⅔ cups (660 mL) Sesame Seasoned Coleslaw (p. 122)
1 cup (250 mL) Green Cashew Coconut Curry Sauce (p. 65)
½ cup (125 mL) chopped red bell pepper
¼ cup (60 mL) sliced Jerusalem artichokes
1 cup (250 mL) broccoli florets

1. In a mixing bowl, toss all ingredients together thoroughly.

Makes 4–6 servings.

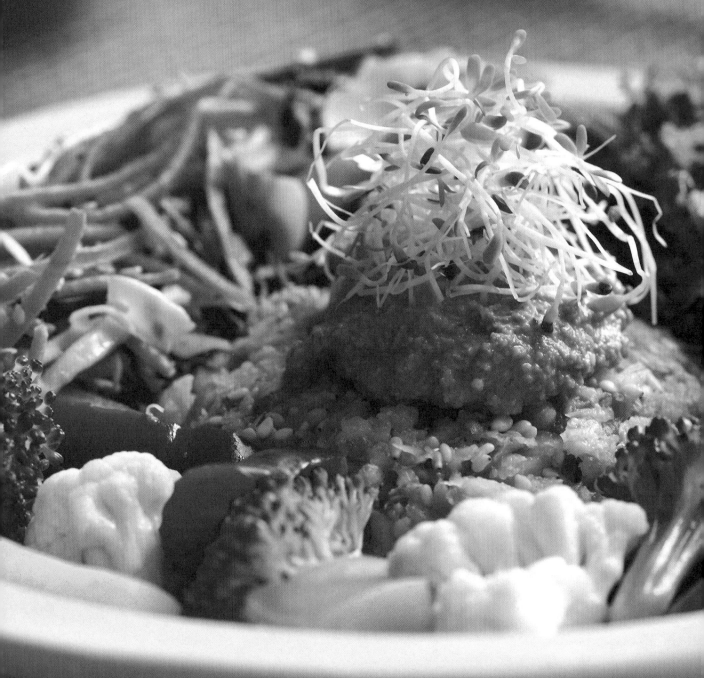

Oh My Gado Gado Nice Bowl

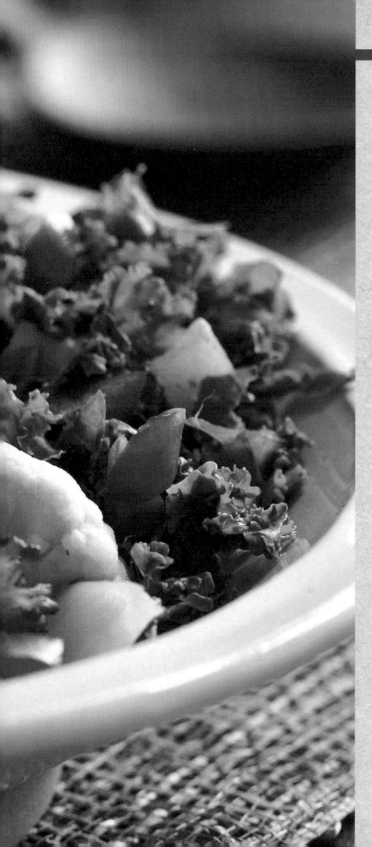

This is a toast to my friend, Long Life!

1 cup (250 mL) Ryce (p. 126)
½ cup (125 mL) Tossed and Tenderized Deep
 Greens (p. 134)
¾ cup (185 mL) Sesame Seasoned Coleslaw
 (p. 122)
¾ cup (185 mL) Gado Marinated Veggies
 (p. 124)
⅓ cup (80 mL) Oh My Gado Peanut Sauce
 (p. 68)
¾ cup (185 mL) sprouts (clover, alfalfa,
 sunflower etc.)
1–2 tbsp chopped jungle peanuts

1. In a bowl place a mound of Ryce.

2. Surround Ryce with three sections
 consisting of greens, coleslaw, and
 marinated veggies.

3. Pour peanut sauce over the Ryce.

4. Garnish with sprouts and chopped
 peanuts.

Makes 1 serving.

Falafel Wrap

We first served these on "Fusion Fridays" during Gorilla Food's early days. I remember coming up with the idea of using pumpkin and sunflower seeds in falafel balls and knowing they would be super great even though I hadn't even tried them yet. I give thanks!

1 romaine lettuce leaf
3–4 tbsp Zucchini Hummus (p. 75)
5–6 Falafel Balls (p. 169)
3–4 tbsp Tahini Drizzle (p. 69)
3–4 tbsp Grainless Tabouli (p. 128)

1. Place lettuce leaf on a plate.

2. Spread a layer of hummus over top.

3. Set falafel balls side by side into the hummus.

4. Spread tahini evenly over falafel balls without covering them completely.

5. Spread tabouli evenly over top, leaving other ingredients visible.

6. Serve as an open-face wrap.

Makes 1 serving.

Falafel Balls

Sprouted seed falafel balls! These are inspired by the international Middle Eastern favorite. Falafel balls are great to have around as a tapa, snack, or canapé, to toss into a salad, or for Falafel Wraps (p. 168).

2 cups (500 mL) sunflower seeds
½ cup (125 mL) pumpkin seeds
2 zucchinis
3½ carrots

1 tsp salt
3 tsp ground paprika
2 tbsp + 1 tsp ground cumin
½ cup (125 mL) whole flax seeds

1. Soak sunflower and pumpkin seeds together for 6 hours or overnight and rinse well before using.

2. In a food processor with an s-blade, process soaked seeds to a sticky consistency. Empty into a bowl.

3. In a food processor with an s-blade, process zucchini, carrots, salt, paprika, and cumin. Add to seed mix.

4. In a blender or coffee grinder, grind flax seeds into a powder. Add to the bowl and mix together well.

5. By hand or with an ice cream scooper, form 1-tbsp falafel balls and place on mesh sheets. Dehydrate at 108°F (42°C) for 16–20 hours, until falafel balls are dry on the outside but still moist on the inside.

Makes 60 balls.

Green Taco

You can also serve this leaf-wrap taco with a slice of Veggie Flax Bread (p. 35).

1 romaine lettuce leaf
¼ cup (60 mL) Walnut Chili Pâté (p. 87)
3–4 tbsp Guacamole (p. 78)
¼ cup (60 mL) Salsa (p. 79), lightly strained

1. Place lettuce leaf on a plate.

2. Spread Chili Pâté across center of leaf.

3. Top evenly with guacamole, leaving pâté visible.

4. Top with salsa, leaving guacamole and pâté visible.

5. Fold leaf in half, to resemble a taco shell.

Makes 1 taco.

International Maki

As a vegan, I appreciate Japanese cuisine a lot! This recipe is inspired by traditional Japanese maki (rolled sushi).

1 nori sheet
2 tbsp Salty Mango Concoct (p. 71)
1–2 lettuce leaves
¼ cup (60 mL) Sunny Ginger Pâté (p. 46)
3 red pepper strips (about ½-in [1-cm]) wide
2–3 cucumber strips (about ½-in [1-cm]) wide
2–3 avocado strips (about ½-in [1-cm]) wide
⅓ cup (80 mL) Carrot & Daikon Hemp Seed Toss (p. 118)
½ cup (125 mL) sprouts (alfalfa, clover, sunflower, etc.)

1. On a dry surface, lay out nori sheet. Spread mango over bottom ¼.

2. Cover with lettuce leaves, leaving about 2 in (5 cm) at top of nori sheet uncovered.

3. Fill lettuce with a mounded layer of pâté.

4. Alongside the pâté, place pepper, cucumber, and avocado strips.

5. Top with carrot and daikon mix and add layer of sprouts.

6. With a bowl of water beside you, roll nori sheet up carefully, making sure everything is tight inside. Moisten the top 2-in (5-cm) section of nori sheet as if an envelope. Finish rolling so both sides stick together. Make sure it is sealed, using more water if necessary.

7. Cut into about 8 pieces or leave as full or half wraps.

Makes 1 roll (or 8 pieces).

Ocean Wrap

A savory roll that you can cut into bite-sized pieces or serve as a larger wrap.

1 nori sheet
2 tbsp Salty Mango Concoct (p. 71)
1–2 lettuce leaves
¼ cup (60 mL) Ocean Pâté (p. 82)
2–3 red pepper strips (about ½-in [1-cm]) wide
3 cucumber strips (about ½-in [1-cm]) wide
2–3 avocado strips (about ½-in [1-cm]) wide
⅓ cup (80 mL) Carrot & Daikon Hemp Seed Toss (p. 118)
½ cup (125 mL) sprouts (alfalfa, clover, sunflower, etc.)

1. On a dry surface, lay out nori sheet. Spread mango over bottom ¼.

2. Cover with lettuce leaves, leaving about 2 in (5 cm) at top of nori sheet uncovered.

3. Fill lettuce with a mounded layer of pâté.

4. Alongside the pâté, place pepper, cucumber, and avocado strips.

5. Top with carrot and daikon mix and add layer of sprouts.

6. With a bowl of water beside you, roll nori sheet up carefully, making sure everything is tight inside. Moisten the top 2-in (5-cm) section of nori sheet as if an envelope. Finish rolling so both sides stick together. Make sure it is sealed, using more water if necessary.

7. Cut into about 8 pieces or leave as full or half wraps.

Makes 1 roll (or 8 pieces).

S'weed as Curry Veggie Maki

I first started making these rolls on a trip to Australia, where the locals would tell me, "These rolls are sweet as, mate!" Serve with your choice of dips or dressings.

1½ cups (375 mL) Tossed and Tenderized Deep Greens (p. 134)
¾ cup (185 mL) Sesame Seasoned Coleslaw (p. 122)
3–4 tbsp Green Cashew Coconut Curry Sauce (p. 65)
2 nori sheets

1. In a large bowl, toss the greens and coleslaw with curry sauce.

2. Divide mix in half and distribute evenly on each nori sheet, leaving about 2-in (5 cm) at top of nori sheet uncovered.

3. With a bowl of water beside you, roll nori sheet up carefully, making sure everything is tight inside. Moisten the top 2-in (5-cm) section of nori sheet as if an envelope. Finish rolling so both sides stick together. Make sure it is sealed, using more water if necessary.

4. Cut each roll into 8 pieces.

Makes 2 servings (16 pieces).

Livity Love

Simple pleasures! If you start with great ingredients, you will have great results. Fresh, ripe, and juicy!

1 slice Veggie Flax Bread (p. 35) or Curry Squash Bread (p. 36)
2 tbsp Guacamole (p. 78)
8–10 thin cucumber slices (or more, if made super-thin with a mandoline)
3–4 tomato slices
1 cup (250 mL) sprouts (alfalfa, clover, sunflower, etc.)
1 large lettuce leaf

1. Cut slice of bread into 2 triangles and place them side by side.

2. On each piece, place a dollop of guacamole and spread evenly.

3. On one piece only, place a layer of cucumber slices, then top with tomato slices.

4. Top tomatoes with thick layer of sprouts and cover with lettuce leaf.

5. Cut other piece of bread (with just guacamole on it) in half so that when you place it on top and cut through, the sandwich won't get too squished.

6. Place the two halves of bread on top of lettuce and cut through to the bottom of sandwich.

Makes 1 serving.

Main St. Monkey

A flavorful, filling sandwich full of rich and juicy ingredients.

1 slice Veggie Flax Bread (p. 35) or Curry Squash Bread (p. 36)
2–3 tbsp Monkey Tapenade (p. 77)
2–3 tbsp Guacamole (p. 78)
8–10 thin cucumber slices (or more, if made super-thin with a mandoline)
3 tomato slices
1 cup (250 mL) sprouts (alfalfa, clover, sunflower, etc.)
2 tbsp Zucchini Hummus (p. 75)

1. Cut slice of bread into 2 triangles and place them side by side.

2. On one piece only, layer a dollop of tapenade and spread evenly.

3. Add large dollop of guacamole and spread evenly.

4. Top with layer of cucumber and tomato slices.

5. Add thick layer of sprouts.

6. On other piece of bread, spread a large dollop of hummus evenly. Cut this piece in half so that when you place it on top and cut through, the sandwich won't get too squished.

7. Place the two halves of bread on top and cut through to the bottom of sandwich.

Makes 1 serving.

Sunny Gorilla

A flavorful and lively favorite!

1 slice Veggie Flax Bread (p. 35) or Curry Squash Bread (p. 36)
¼–⅜ cup (60–90 mL) Sunny Ginger Pâté (p. 46)
⅓ cup (80 mL) Guacamole & Greens (p. 135)
8–10 thin cucumber slices (or more, if made super-thin with a mandoline)
1 cup (250 mL) sprouts (alfalfa, clover, sunflower, etc.)
1 lettuce leaf

1. Cut slice of bread into 2 triangles and place them side by side.

2. Cover both halves with pâté.

3. On one piece only, spread dollop of Guacamole & Greens, then add cucumber slices, covering bread entirely.

4. Add layer of sprouts, then top with lettuce leaf.

5. Add thick layer of sprouts.

6. Cut other piece of bread in half so that when you place it on top and cut through, the sandwich won't get too squished.

7. Place the two halves of bread on top and cut through to the bottom of sandwich.

Makes 1 serving.

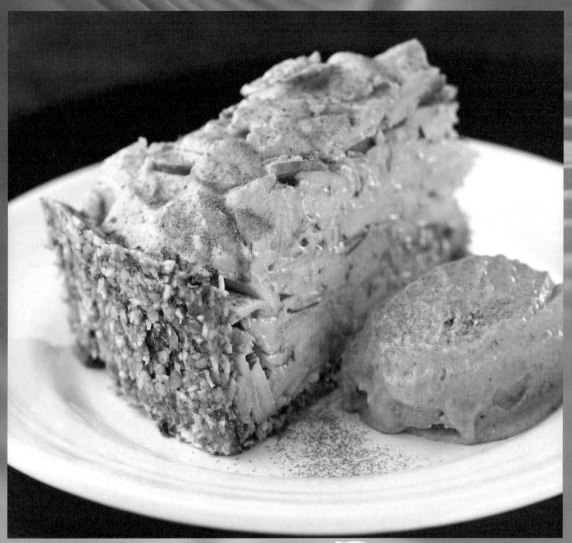

Desserts

Bliss Butterflies

Use beautiful walnut halves so these butterflies live up to their name!

1 recipe Vanilla Fudge (p. 187)
¼–⅓ cup (60–80 mL) Golden Caramel (p. 183)
12–16 walnut halves

1. With a cookie cutter, stamp a flower or any other shape into the fudge. You can press together any leftover chocolate and cut out 1 or 2 more shapes.)

2. Roll 1 tsp caramel into a ball for each piece of fudge.

3. Press walnut half into caramel, then squish it down to stick in center of fudge.

Makes 12–16 pieces.

Chocolate Cherry Bombs

I love the ginger and the little bits of chewy dried cherries in these truffles.

⅜ cup (90 mL) shredded cacao butter
¾ cup (185 mL) cacao nibs
½ cup (125 mL) cashews
16 dates, pitted
¼ tsp vanilla powder
1¼ tsp dried, powdered ginger
½ cup (125 mL) chopped dried cherries
2 tsp hemp seeds

1. Melt cacao butter in a bowl using the warmth of the dehydrator at 108°F (42°C) or by floating a metal bowl containing cacao butter in another bowl of hot tap water (like a double boiler).

2. In a coffee grinder, grind cacao nibs to a fine powder.

3. In a food processor with an s-blade, blend cashews to a creamy, buttery consistency. Place in a bowl.

4. In a food processor with an s-blade, process melted cacao butter, dates, vanilla, and ginger to a toffee-like consistency.

5. Add cacao powder and blend until smooth and combined well.

6. Add dried cherries and hemp seeds and blend until just mixed. Add cashew butter and mix well.

7. Hand-roll 1-tbsp portions into balls and chill to set (3–4 hours).

Makes approximately 16 balls.

Chocolate Fudge

This recipe takes me back to the start of a serious joy in making chocolate!

⅜ cup (90 mL) shredded cacao butter
¾ cup (185 mL) cacao nibs
17 dates, pitted

1. Melt cacao butter in a bowl using the warmth of the dehydrator at 108°F (42°C) or by floating a metal bowl containing cacao butter in another bowl of hot tap water (like a double boiler).

2. In a coffee grinder, grind cacao nibs to a fine powder.

3. In a food processor with an s-blade, blend dates and melted cacao butter until well mixed.

4. Add cacao powder and blend until smooth and combined well.

5. Form a mound of chocolate fudge onto a ParaFlexx sheet and lay another sheet over top of it. Press the slab flat using a rolling pin or press down on it with a cutting board.

6. Chill to set (3–4 hours).

7. Slice into 12–16 squares.

Makes 12–16 fudge squares.

Chocolate Nut Log

Last second, rushing out the door to an event, chocolate craving, oh no, not much time, a-ha! Food processor, ingredients, good vibrations, pen, paper, here, blessed!

¾ cup (185 mL) almonds
3 tbsp hemp seeds
¾ cup (185 mL) raisins
¼ cup (60 mL) sesame seeds
1 tbsp cacao butter
3 tbsp coconut oil

2½ tbsp carob powder
½ cup + 2 tbsp (135 mL) cacao powder
½ tbsp maca powder
½ tsp vanilla powder
16 dates, pitted

1. In a food processor with an s-blade, process all ingredients until mixture starts to stick together.

2. Remove from processor and roll into a log form.

3. Chill to set (3–4 hours) before slicing into rounds.

Makes 12–16 servings.

Jungle Peanut Butter Cups

I often over-indulge on these because they're so good! This recipe makes one serving, but you can make as many as you would like.

1 tbsp Vanilla Fudge (p. 187)
2 tsp Jungle Peanut Butter (p. 91)

1. Portion and press fudge into semisphere or saucer-shaped latex form. Press flat and chill to set (3–4 hours), then pop out of the mold.

2. Put peanut butter in a pastry bag and squeeze rosebud onto chocolate.

Makes 1 JPB cup.

Orange Essence Truffles

A creamy, dense truffle with a citrus essence.

1 tbsp orange zest
¼ cup (60 mL) shredded cacao butter
¾ cups (185 mL) cacao nibs
17 dates, pitted

1 tbsp coconut oil
2 tsp vanilla powder
1 pinch salt
2–3 tbsp cacao powder (for dusting)

1. Dehydrate orange zest on mesh sheets at 108°F (42°C) 8–12 hours or overnight.

2. In a blender, process dried zest to a powder.

3. Melt cacao butter in a bowl using the warmth of the dehydrator at 108°F (42°C) or by floating a metal bowl containing cacao butter in another bowl containing hot tap water (like a double boiler).

4. In a coffee grinder, grind cacao nibs to a fine powder.

5. In a food processor with an s-blade, combine dates with melted cacao butter, orange zest, oil, vanilla, and salt. Process to a toffee-like consistency.

6. Add cacao powder and blend until thoroughly mixed and toffee-like again.

7. Using 1 tbsp of mixture per truffle, hand-roll into balls and then roll in cacao powder.

Makes approximately 16 truffles.

Golden Caramel

One day, I set out to make white chocolate but ended up with a golden surprise. Use this in Bliss Butterflies (p. 178).

3 tbsp shredded cacao butter
8 dates, pitted

1. Melt cacao butter in a bowl using the warmth of the dehydrator at 108°F (42°C) or by floating a metal bowl containing cacao butter in another bowl of hot tap water (like a double boiler).

2. In a food processor with an s-blade, blend dates and melted cacao butter to a toffee-like consistency.

3. Leave at room temperature to set and to allow for optimum spreadability.

Makes ⅔ cup (160 mL).

Maca Chocoroons

These chewy treats are nice to have around—if you can keep them around!

¼ cup (60 mL) shredded cacao butter
¾–1 cup (185–250 mL) cacao nibs
18 dates, pitted
1½ cups (310 mL) coconut flakes
2½ tsp maca powder

1. Melt cacao butter in a bowl using the warmth of the dehydrator at 108°F (42°C) or by floating a metal bowl containing cacao butter in another bowl of hot tap water (like a double boiler).

2. In a coffee grinder, grind cacao nibs to a fine powder.

3. In a food processor with an s-blade, blend the dates and the melted cacao butter until combined well.

4. Add cacao powder and process until thoroughly mixed.

5. In a bowl, toss coconut flakes with maca powder.

6. Add cacao and date purée to coconut and maca mix and combine thoroughly by hand.

7. Hand-form 2-tbsp portions into balls or haystacks and chill to set (3–4 hours).

Makes 16 chocoroons.

Protein Orbs Pre-soak

You can make these with dry nuts too (i.e., don't soak them); if so, they can be stored longer.

1 cup (250 mL) walnuts
¼ cup (60 mL) pumpkin seeds
¼ cup (60 mL) hemp seeds
2 tsp hemp protein powder
½ cup (125 mL) coconut flakes

¼ cup (60 mL) cacao nibs
7 dates, pitted
1 tbsp coconut oil
½ cup (125 mL) coconut flakes (for rolling orbs in)

1. In a bowl, soak walnuts and seeds for 4 hours; rinse well with fresh water before using.

2. In a food processor with an s-blade, process walnuts and seeds until they are coarse but a little sticky. Place in a large bowl.

3. Add hemp seeds, hemp protein, and ½ cup (125 mL) coconut flakes and combine well.

4. In a coffee grinder, grind cacao nibs to a fine powder.

5. In a food processor with an s-blade, process dates and oil to a smooth and toffee-like consistency. Add to nut and seed mix.

6. Add cacao nib powder and mix by hand until well blended.

7. Form balls with 2-tbsp scoops, then roll in ½ cup (125 mL) coconut flakes to finish.

Makes 18 orbs.

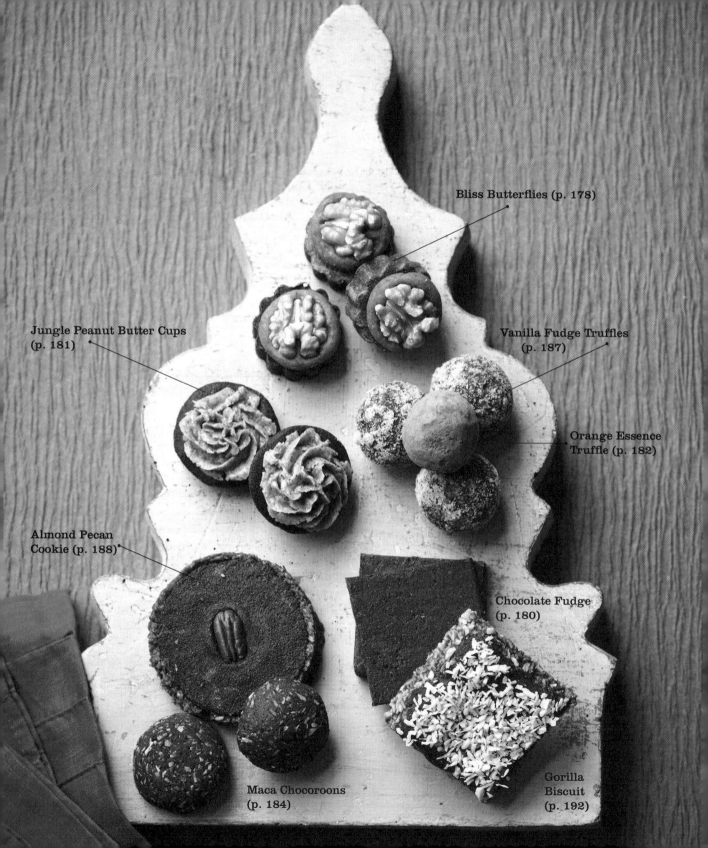

Bliss Butterflies (p. 178)

Jungle Peanut Butter Cups
(p. 181)

Vanilla Fudge Truffles
(p. 187)

Orange Essence
Truffle (p. 182)

Almond Pecan
Cookie (p. 188)

Chocolate Fudge
(p. 180)

Maca Chocoroons
(p. 184)

Gorilla
Biscuit
(p. 192)

Vanilla Fudge

This is a base recipe for many different chocolate options (see Step 6 below). Experiment with different varieties of vanilla to find the kind you like best.

¾ cups (185 mL) shredded cacao butter
¼ cup (60 mL) cacao nibs
17 dates, pitted
1½ tsp vanilla powder
1 tbsp coconut oil

1. Melt cacao butter in a bowl in the warmth of the dehydrator at 108°F (42°C) or by floating a metal bowl containing cacao butter in another bowl containing hot tap water (like a double boiler).

2. In a coffee grinder, grind cacao nibs to a fine powder.

3. In a food processor with an s-blade, process dates with melted cacao butter, vanilla, and oil to a smooth toffee-like consistency.

4. Add cacao powder and process until thoroughly mixed and toffee-like again.

5. Flatten between 2 ParaFlexx sheets with a rolling pin or by pressing with a cutting board.

6. Chill to set (3–4 hours) before cutting into shapes (see Bliss Butterflies, p. 178). You can also work with it while the chocolate is still soft or utilize a latex mold (see Jungle Peanut Butter Cups, p. 181), or roll it into a truffle.

Makes approximately 12–16 pieces.

Almond Pecan Cookies

This recipe evolved out of the Peace Cookies (p. 195). My favorite way to enjoy these is to frost them with Chocolate Fudge (p. 180).

1⅓ cups (315 mL) almonds
1 cup (250 mL) sunflower seeds
1 cup (250 mL) pecans
9 dates, pitted
2 tbsp coconut oil
1½ tbsp grated cacao butter
2½ bananas

1. In a bowl, soak almonds, sunflower seeds, and pecans together overnight (8–12 hours) and rinse well before using.

2. In a food processor with an s-blade, blend dates, oil, and cacao butter together to a toffee-like consistency.

3. Add bananas and blend until smooth and combined well. Pour into a large bowl.

4. In a food processor, process nuts and seeds to a sticky consistency. Add to dates and banana mix and combine well by hand.

5. Form ⅓-cup (80-mL) cookies on mesh sheets and dry overnight at 108°F (42°C). Flip them over and continue to dehydrate at same temperature for another 24–48 hours, depending on desired texture: soft and chewy or crunchy.

Makes 18 cookies.

Cinnamon Almond Crunch Cookies

I like to snack on the batter while making these cookies. I think they're more nutritious than most breakfast cereals, so I say it's okay to have them for breakfast!

1¼ cup (310 mL) sunflower seeds
1 cup (250 mL) almonds
½ cup (125 mL) pumpkin seeds
2 cups (500 mL) coconut flakes
1⅓ cups (315 mL) raisins
½ cup (125 mL) goji berries
8 dates, pitted

1 tsp ground cinnamon
⅓ tsp salt
1⅓ tbsp coconut oil
2 bananas, sliced
1⅔ cups (410 mL) cored and chopped
  apples

1. In a bowl, soak seeds overnight and rinse well before using. Sunflower seeds and almonds can be soaked together, but the pumpkin seeds should be soaked separately.

2. In a separate bowl, soak raisins and goji berries for at least 2 hours.

3. In a food processor with an s-blade, coarsely process sunflower seeds and almonds just until sticky but still a little coarse. Add to a large bowl with pumpkin seeds, coconut flakes, raisins, and goji berries.

4. In a food processor with an s-blade, process dates, cinnamon, salt, and coconut oil to a toffee-like consistency.

5. In a food processor, process bananas to a smooth sauce. Add to the bowl.

6. In a food processor, purée apples, then add to the bowl and mix to combine well.

7. Form ⅓-cup (80-mL) cookies on mesh sheets and dehydrate at 108°F (42°C) for 12–18 hours. Flip them over and continue to dehydrate at same temperature for another 24–30 hours.

Makes 18 cookies.

Choco Halva

For a while I was eating so much of this treat that I started to get hot flashes. You'll have to eat a lot for that to happen, though!

½ cup (125 mL) cacao nibs
2 cups (500 mL) sesame seeds
10 dates, pitted
2 tbsp coconut oil

1. In a coffee grinder, grind cacao nibs to a fine powder.

2. In a food processor with an s-blade, process sesame seeds into tahini. Place in a bowl and set aside.

3. In a food processor with an s-blade, blend dates and coconut oil to a toffee-like consistency.

4. Add cacao powder and blend until fully mixed.

5. Add tahini back in and process until evenly blended.

6. Press mixture into a springform pan and chill to set (3–4 hours).

7. Cut into 8 triangular slices.

Makes 8 servings.

Golden Halva

Simplicity at its best!

2½ cups (625 mL) sesame seeds
11 dates, pitted

1. In a food processor with an s-blade, blend sesame seeds into tahini. Set aside in a bowl.

2. In a food processor with an s-blade, blend dates to a toffee-like consistency.

3. Add tahini back in and mix well until evenly blended.

4. Press flat in a 10-in (25-cm) springform pan and chill to set (3–4 hours).

5. Cut into 8 triangular slices.

Makes 8 serving.

Gorilla Biscuits

These sweet treats were named as a tribute to the great NYC punk band.

4 dates, pitted
1 tbsp coconut oil
1 tsp ground cinnamon
9 bananas, sliced
4½ cups (1 L + 125 mL) coconut flakes

1. In a food processor with an s-blade, process dates, coconut oil, and cinnamon to a toffee-like consistency.

2. Add a few banana slices to thin out the paste, then add more to thin it out further. Pour into a large bowl.

3. In a food processor with an s-blade, blend rest of bananas, in batches, into a purée. Pour into the bowl, stirring evenly into date mix.

4. Add coconut flakes and mix thoroughly by hand.

5. Spread mixture onto 1 or 2 mesh dehydrator sheets, ¼–½-in (½–1-cm) thick.

6. Stamp out shapes with a cookie cutter or score 6 x 6-in (15 x 15-cm) squares with the dull side of a knife.

7. Dehydrate at 108°F (42°C) for 36 hours. Flip them over and continue to dehydrate at same temperature for another 24 hours or until fully dry.

Makes 24–36 biscuits.

Super Star Bars Pre-soak

Why not make your own whole food energy bars instead of buying them and throwing away the packaging? These are great for traveling or as an after-exercise snack. You can add any additional super-food and protein powders to your taste.

½ cup (125 mL) almonds
1 cup (250 mL) sunflower seeds
⅓ cup (80 mL) pecans
¼ cup (60 mL) goji berries
⅓ cup (80 mL) chopped dried apricots
4 dates, pitted

¼ tsp salt
1 tbsp coconut oil
1 apple, cored
2 bananas
2 tbsp hemp protein powder
1 tsp maca powder

1. In a bowl, soak almonds, seeds, and pecans in water for 8–12 hours or overnight and rinse well before using.

2. In a separate bowl, soak goji berries and apricots for 1 hour.

3. In a food processor with an s-blade, process almonds, seeds, and pecans until minced and sticky. Set aside in a bowl.

4. In a food processor with an s-blade, process dates, salt, and coconut oil to a toffee-like consistency.

5. Add apple, bananas, hemp protein and maca powder, and purée. Add to bowl.

6. Add goji berries and apricots and mix to combine well.

7. Spread mixture ¼–½-in (½–1 cm) thick on ParaFlexx sheets and dehydrate at 108°F (42°C) for 12–16 hours.

8. Flip over onto mesh sheets and continue to dehydrate at the same temperature for another 24 hours or until dry.

Makes 12 bars.

Orange Walnut Spice Cookies

After many years of making these, I still love eating them. Although I leave them chewy, they remind me of my grandpa's gingersnap cookies that he always had around (even though they contain no ginger).

3 cups (750 mL) walnuts
1 cup (250 mL) sunflower seeds
1 cup (250 mL) raisins
15 dates, pitted

3½ tsp ground cinnamon
½ tsp ground nutmeg
1½ tsp ground allspice
¾ cup (185 mL) orange juice

1. In a bowl, soak walnuts and sunflower seeds overnight or for at least 6 hours and rinse well before using.

2. In a separate bowl, soak raisins for 1–2 hours.

3. In a food processor with an s-blade, process dates, spices, and orange juice into a paste. Set aside in a large bowl.

4. In a food processor with an s-blade, process nuts and seeds to a coarse paste and add to date mix.

5. Add raisins and mix by hand until combined well.

6. Form ⅓-cup (80-mL) cookies and place onto mesh sheets and dehydrate at 108°F (42°C) for 12–18 hours. Flip them over and continue to dehydrate at the same temperature for another 12–18 hours, until they have attained desired consistency.

Makes 16 cookies.

Peace Cookies Pre-soak

There's nothing like sweet, fresh pecans, especially in these cookies!

1½ cups (375 mL) pecans
¾ cup (185 mL) almonds
8 dates, pitted
3 tbsp coconut oil

1. Soak nuts for 8–12 hours or overnight and rinse well before using.

2. In a food processor with an s-blade, blend dates and coconut oil to a toffee-like consistency. Set aside in a bowl.

3. In a food processor with an s-blade, process nuts to a coarse but sticky texture. Add to date mix and combine well by hand.

4. Portion into ¼-cup (60-mL) scoops and form into wide flat cookies on a mesh sheet and dehydrate at 108°F (42°C) for 12–16 hours. Flip them over and continue to dehydrate at same temperature for another 12–36 hours, until they have attained desired texture.

Makes 9 cookies.

Rawk Luva

This one goes out to Maria!

Pastry Sheets:
2 cups (500 mL) walnuts
4 dates, pitted
¼ cup (60 mL) flax seeds

¼ tsp ground cinnamon
1 cup (250 mL) water

1. In a bowl, soak walnuts for 4 hours or overnight and rinse well before using.

2. In a blender, process all ingredients until smooth.

3. Divide batter between 2 ParaFlexx sheets and spread evenly out to the edges Dehydrate at 108°F (42°C) for 8–12 hours or overnight.

4. Flip them over onto mesh sheets and continue to dehydrate at same temperature for another 4 hours.

Cream Filling:
1½ cups (375 mL) walnuts
7 dates, pitted
½ tsp powdered vanilla

¼ tsp ground cinnamon
2 tbsp lemon juice

1. In a bowl, soak walnuts for 4 hours or overnight and rinse well before using.

2. In a food processor with an s-blade, process dates, vanilla, cinnamon, and lemon juice into a paste.

3. Add walnuts and process until smooth.

To assemble:
1 cup (250 mL) walnuts, finely chopped
2 Pastry Sheets (above)
1¾ cups (415 mL, or 1 recipe) Cream
  Filling (above)

1. Spread Cream Filling evenly on the
   two pastry sheets, out to the edges.

2. Sprinkle walnuts over top.

3. Cut each sheet into 4 strips
   (you will have 8 in total).

4. Layer 7 strips on top of one another
   with frosting side up on top, and
   last strip with frosting facing down.

5. Press lightly on stack, then carefully cut into triangles or diamonds
   (like baklava, the Greek and Middle
   Eastern treat).

Makes approximately 8 servings.

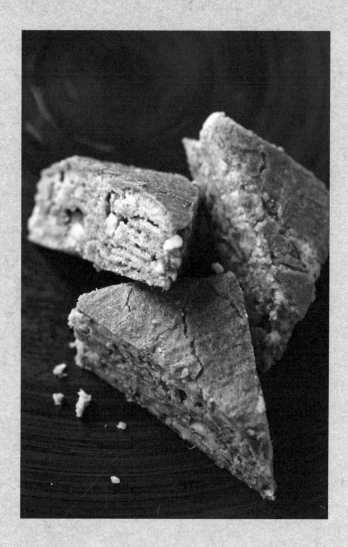

Two Berry Goodness Cashew Ice Cream

Sweet, frosty, fruity, and creamy—vegan ice cream is the best!

1 cup (250 mL) cashews
2 tbsp goji berries
6 dates, pitted
⅜ cup (90 mL) coconut oil

2¼ cups (530 mL) chopped strawberries
½ tsp powdered vanilla
1 cup (250 mL) water

1. In a blender, process all ingredients until oil has melted and mixture is smooth.

2. Pour into a bowl and freeze, or churn in an ice cream maker according to manufacturer's directions.

Makes 2–4 servings.

Chocolate Coconut Ice Cream

It's so hard to have only a little of this ice cream—it's like being a kid again! Young coconuts are white and cone-shaped; they can be found in many Asian grocery and health food stores. The flesh of the coconut gets thicker and dryer as it matures; when still young, it's soft, and the coconut water is sweet and refreshing.

1 cup (250 mL) fresh young coconut "meat"
1¾ cups (415 mL) young coconut water

½ cup (125 mL) cacao nibs
7 dates, pitted
¼ cup (60 mL) coconut oil

1. In a blender, process all ingredients until oil has melted and mixture is smooth.

2. Pour into a bowl and freeze, or churn in an ice cream maker according to manufacturer's directions.

Makes 2–4 servings.

Chocolate Hempcicles

These have been a summertime hit when we've served them at the Mr. Fresh booth at music festivals over the years.

½ cup (125 mL) cacao nibs
9 dates, pitted
⅜ cup (90 mL) hemp seeds

½ cup (125 mL) coconut oil
2 tbsp cacao butter
1¼ cups (310 mL) water

1. In blender, process all ingredients until oil has melted and mixture is smooth.

2. Pour into popsicle molds.

3. Place a popsicle stick into each mold and freeze.

Makes approximately 6 servings.

Lemon Avocado Ice Cream

Let this refreshing treat soften slightly before serving.

2 bananas
1½ tbsp chia seeds
8 dates, pitted
⅜ cup (90 mL) coconut oil

3 avocados
¾ tsp spirulina
½ cup (125 mL) lemon juice

1. In a blender, process all ingredients until oil has melted and mixture is smooth.

2. Pour into a bowl and freeze, or churn in an ice cream maker according to manufacturer's directions.

Makes 2½ cups (625 mL).

Orange Avocado Ice Cream

Sweet subtle flavors with a creamy, smooth texture. Let soften slightly before serving.

2½ bananas
½ cup (125 mL) coconut oil
11 dates, pitted

1 vanilla bean
2–3 avocados
1½ tsp orange zest

1. In a blender, process all ingredients until oil has melted and mixture is smooth.

2. Add avocado and blend until combined well.

3. Pour into a bowl and place in freezer until frozen (3–4 hours).

Makes 2½ cups (625 mL).

Peach Coconut Ice Cream

I've noticed that sweet peaches have a much more amazing flavor when they're ripened while still on the tree.

2 cups (500 mL) young coconut meat
3 tbsp coconut oil
3 dates, pitted

2½ cups (625 mL) chopped peaches
½ cups (125 mL) chopped strawberries
½ banana

1. In a blender, process all ingredients until oil has melted and mixture is smooth.

2. Pour into a bowl and freeze, or churn in an ice cream maker according to manufacturer's directions.

Makes 5 cups (1¼ L).

Strawberry Cashew Ice Cream

The better the strawberries, the better the ice cream. Praise to creamy cashews!

1 cup (250 mL) cashews
7 dates, pitted
2½ cups (625 mL) strawberries

½ tsp powdered vanilla
⅜ cup (90 mL) coconut oil
¾ cup (185 mL) water

1. In a blender, process all ingredients until oil has melted and mixture is smooth.

2. Pour into a bowl and freeze, or churn in an ice cream maker according to manufacturer's directions.

Makes 4 cups (1 L).

Dark Cherry Ice Cream Cake

Ice cream + cake = giving thanks!

Cake base:
3½ cups (830 mL) coconut flakes
8 dates, pitted

1. In a food processor with an s-blade, blend until dates and coconut are finely ground and stick together.

2. Press mixture flat and evenly across the bottom of a 10-in (25-cm) springform pan.

3. Chill to set (3–4 hours).

Ice Cream Filling:
⅔ cup (160 mL) pitted dried cherries
6 bananas
6 dates, pitted
⅜ cup (90 mL) coconut oil
1½ cups (375 mL) cashews
⅜ tsp vanilla powder

1. In a bowl, soak cherries for 3–4 hours.

2. In a blender, blend all ingredients until smooth.

3. Pour and spread over top of cake base in springform pan and freeze to set.

Makes 1 (10-in [25-cm]) cake.

Basic Pie Crust

Can you imagine all the new fillings you can try in this crust? For a start, try those on pages 206-08!

⅔ cup (160 mL) almonds
1 cup (250 mL) sunflower seeds
5–6 dates, pitted

2 tbsp coconut oil
¼ tsp salt
1⅓ cups (315 mL) shredded coconut

1. In a bowl, soak almonds and sunflower seeds for ½–4 hours and rinse well before using.

2. In a food processor with an s-blade, pulse-grind nuts and seeds until sticky. Place in a bowl and set aside.

3. In a food processor with an s-blade, blend dates, coconut oil, and salt until smooth. Add to bowl.

4. Add shredded coconut and mix well by hand.

5. Press dough evenly into bottom of 10-in (25-cm) springform pan ¾ of the way up the sides.

Makes 1 (10-in [25-cm]) pie.

Pre-soak

Apple Pie

This is a fresh take on Grandma's classic!

Crust:
⅓ cup (80 mL) almonds
⅔ cup (160 mL) sunflower seeds
4 dates, pitted
¼ tsp salt

1 tbsp coconut oil
1⅓ cups (315 mL) coconut flakes
1 cup (250 mL) cashews

1. In a bowl, soak almonds and seeds for ½–2 hours or overnight and rinse well before using. To let them sprout longer, just rinse every 8–12 hours for a couple of days.

2. In a food processor with an s-blade, pulse almonds and seeds until sticky but still a little crunchy. Set aside in a bowl.

3. In a food processor with an s-blade, process dates, salt, and coconut oil until smooth. Add to bowl along with shredded coconut flakes.

4. In a food processor with an s-blade, pulse-grind cashews until not quite powdered but crumbly. Add to bowl and combine well by hand.

5. Press dough evenly into 10-in (25-cm) springform pan and chill to set (3–4 hours) while you make the filling.

Filling:
7–8 apples, cored
3½–4 bananas
½ cup (125 mL) chopped strawberries
½ cup (125 mL) coconut oil
½ tsp ground cinnamon
¼ tsp ground nutmeg
3 dates, pitted
½–¾ tsp ground cinnamon
  (for garnish)

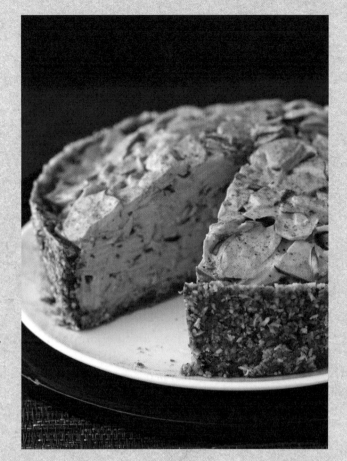

1. In a food processor with a slicer disc, slice apples thinly. Set aside in a bowl.

2. In a blender, process bananas, strawberries, coconut oil, cinnamon, nutmeg, and dates until oil has melted. Pour over apples and mix thoroughly.

3. Add apple mixture to pie crust and chill (3–4 hours), until set.

4. Remove from the springform pan and carefully slide onto a plate.

5. Dust the top of the pie with cinnamon.

Makes 1 (10-in [25-cm]) pie.

Blueberry Mango Fruit Pie

Loving the summertime blues!

Crust:
1 recipe Basic Pie Crust (p. 203)

Filling:
1½–2 cups (375–500 mL) dried
  mangos
1⅓ cups (315 mL) water
5–6 bananas
3 dates, pitted
¾–⅞ cup (185–210 mL) coconut oil
2¼ cups (530 mL) blueberries

1½ cups (375 mL) blueberries,
  for layering
½ cup (125 mL) blueberries,
  for garnish
2–4 tbsp shredded coconut, for
  garnish

1. In a bowl, soak dried mangos in water for ½–1 hour. Reserve soaking water.

2. In a blender, process mangos with reserved soaking water until smooth. Set aside in a bowl.

3. In blender, process bananas, dates, and coconut oil until smooth.

4. Add 2¼ cups (530 mL) blueberries and blend until smooth. Stir into mango purée.

5. Pour ⅓ of filling into pie crust, then layer 1½ blueberries onto top.

6. Pour rest of filling over top of the berries and chill to set (3–4 hours).

7. Garnish with more blueberries and shredded coconut.

Makes 1 (10-in [25-cm]) pie.

Blueberry Peach Pie

This pie is so summery and juicy! There's just a short time each year when the fruits are in season to enjoy this one.

Crust:
1 recipe Basic Pie Crust (p. 203)

Filling:
4 dates, pitted
⅝ cup (150 mL) coconut oil
¼ tsp vanilla powder
3½–4 bananas

7–8 cups (1¾–2 L) sliced peaches
5 cups (1¼ L) blueberries
peach slices, for garnish
blueberries, for garnish

1. In a blender, process dates, coconut oil, vanilla powder, and bananas until oil is incorporated and mixture is smooth.

2. Arrange ½ of the peaches over pie crust.

3. Pour ¼ of date-banana sauce over peaches. Swirl pan a bit to let sauce fill in the cracks.

4. Layer ½ of the blueberries over top.

5. Pour another ¼ of date-banana sauce over blueberries, then top with rest of peaches.

6. Add another ¼ of the date-banana sauce and top with rest of blueberries.

7. Pour rest of date-banana sauce on top of blueberries.

8. Garnish with a fruit decoration of your choosing. (I use a peach slice and a couple of blueberries on each piece or arrange peaches and blueberries in a mandala design.)

9. Chill to set (3–4 hours).

Makes 1 (10-in [25-cm]) pie.

Other options:
a) Portion filling into bowls with cobbler crust (layering in the same method as the pie). Chill to set (3–4 hours).
b) Pour banana cream over a bowl of chopped peaches and blueberries and stir. Serve chilled.

Desserts

Chocolate Hemp Seed Pie

This was a divine gift—one of those times when I made it, loved it from the first bite, and never tweaked it once.

Crust:
1 recipe Basic Pie Crust (p. 203)

Filling:
⅞ cup (210 mL) cacao nibs
17 dates, pitted
¾ cup (185 mL) hemp seeds
¼ cup (60 mL) + 3 tbsp coconut oil

¼ cup (60 mL) cacao butter
2⅝ cups (650 mL) water
2 tbsp coconut flakes, for garnish
2 tbsp cacao nibs, for garnish

1. In a blender, place all ingredients and blend until oil is incorporated and mixture is smooth.

2. Pour into pie crust and refrigerate to set (3–4 hours).

3. Carefully remove from springform pan and slide pie onto a large plate.

4. Garnish with sprinkles of coconut flakes and cacao nibs.

Makes 1 (10-in [25-cm]) pie.

Coconut Cream Pie

This pie has always been on Gorilla Food's secret-special-request menu because the young coconuts are usually not organic, and we don't usually use them for that reason. I love this one, though; it's so simple!

Crust:
2½ cups (625 mL) coconut flakes	2 tbsp coconut oil
9 dates, pitted	¼ tsp salt

1. In a food processor with an s-blade, process coconut flakes to an oily flour texture. Set aside in a bowl.

2. In a food processor with an s-blade, blend dates, oil, and salt to a toffee-like consistency.

3. Add coconut flour back in and process until combined well.

4. Press dough into a 10-in (25-cm) springform pan and chill to set (3–4 hours) while you make the filling.

Filling:
3 cups (750 mL) young coconut meat	1 tbsp + 2 tsp lemon juice
13 dates, pitted	¼ tsp salt
¾ cup (185 mL) coconut oil	1 cup (250 mL) coconut water

1. In a blender, process all ingredients until oil is incorporated and mixture is smooth. Pour into pie crust and chill to set (3–4 hours).

Makes 1 (10-in [25-cm]) pie.

Lemon Avocado Pie

This pie—so fresh, light, and creamy—has long been a hit at Gorilla Food.

Crust:

2 cups (500 mL) coconut flakes

1 cup (250 mL) Brazil nuts

9 dates, pitted

2 tbsp coconut oil

1. In a food processor with an s-blade, process coconut and Brazil nuts to an oily flour texture. Set aside in a bowl.

2. In a food processor with an s-blade, blend dates and coconut oil to a toffee-like consistency.

3. Add nut mix back in and process until combined well.

4. Press dough into a 10-in (25-cm) springform pan and chill to set (3–4 hours) while you make the filling.

Filling:

16 dates, pitted

3½–4 bananas

3 tbsp chia seeds

¾ cup (185 mL) coconut oil

5–7 avocados

1½ tsp spirulina

⅞ cup (210 mL) lemon juice

1. In a food processor with an s-blade, process dates to a toffee-like consistency.

2. In blender, process bananas, chia seeds, and oil until oil has melted.

3. Combine both mixes in a food processor to thin out and dissolve dates.

4. Add avocado and spirulina and combine until very creamy. Add lemon juice and keep processing until combined well.

5. Pour into pie crust and chill to set (3–4 hours).

Makes 1 (10-in [25-cm]) pie.

Pumpkin Pie

Giving thanks every day!

Crust:
½ cup (125 mL) Brazil nuts
½ cup (125 mL) pecans
2 cups (500 mL) coconut flakes

9 dates, pitted
2 tbsp coconut oil

1. In a food processor with an s-blade, process nuts and coconut flakes until oily and flour-like. Empty into a bowl and set aside.

2. In a food processor, blend dates and oil to a toffee-like consistency.

3. Add nut and coconut mix back in and process until combined well.

4. Press flat and evenly into 10-in (25-cm) springform pan and chill to set (3–4 hours) before filling.

Filling:
6 dates, pitted
¾ cups (185 mL) coconut oil
2¾ tsp pumpkin pie spices (cinnamon, ginger, nutmeg, allspice)

3½–4 bananas
4 cups (1 L) pumpkin, cut into 1–2-in (2½–5-cm) cubes

1. In a blender, process dates, oil, spices, and bananas until oil has melted and mixture is smooth.

2. Add pumpkin and blend until smooth.

3. Pour into pie crust and chill to set (3–4 hours).

Makes 1 (10-in [25-cm]) pie.

Cheezcake Crust

This can be used as the base for any cheezcake.

2 cups (500 mL) coconut flakes
8 dates, pitted

1. In a food processor with an s-blade, blend until dates and coconut stick together.

2. Press flat and evenly across bottom of a 10-in (25-cm) springform pan.

3. Chill to set (3–4 hours).

Makes 1 (10-in [25-cm]) pie.

Blueberry Cheezcake

The sharper the food-processor blade, the creamier this will be. You can also make it in a blender.

Crust:
1 recipe Cheezcake Crust (p. 212)

Filling:
9 dates, pitted
2 tbsp coconut oil
1½ cups (375 mL) coconut flakes
4 cups (1 L) cashews

4½ cups (1 L + 125 mL) blueberries
½ cup (125 mL) blueberries, for garnish
2–4 tbsp shredded coconut, for garnish
2–4 tbsp cashews, for garnish

1. In a food processor with an s-blade, blend dates and oil to a toffee-like consistency.

2. Add coconut flakes and cashews and blend until buttery.

3. Add blueberries and blend until smooth.

4. Press mixture into pie crust. Garnish with berries, shredded coconut, and cashews, then chill to set (3–4 hours).

5. Remove from pan and decorate the sides with additional cashews.

Makes 1 (10-in [25-cm]) pie.

Strawberry Cheezcake

Naturally sweet, naturally colored, naturally beautiful.

Crust:
1½ cups (375 mL) cashews
1½ cups (375 mL) coconut flakes
9 dates, pitted

2 tbsp coconut oil
⅜ tsp salt

1. In a food processor with an s-blade, blend all ingredients until combined well and dates are well-minced; the mixture should stick together.

2. Press flat and evenly across the bottom of a 10-in (25-cm) springform pan and chill to set (3–4 hours) before filling.

Filling:
8 dates, pitted
3 tbsp coconut oil
4 cups (1 L) cashews
½ cup (125 mL) orange juice

1¾ cups (415 mL) chopped strawberries
handful sliced strawberries
handful cashews

1. In a food processor with an s-blade, blend dates and oil to a toffee-like consistency.

2. Add cashews and process until buttery.

3. Add strawberries and orange juice and process until smooth.

4. Pour into pie crust. Garnish with strawberries and cashews and chill to set (3–4 hours).

5. Remove from springform pan and decorate the sides with additional cashews.

Makes 1 (10-in [25-cm]) pie.

Persimmon Cheezcake

I miss persimmon season as soon as it's over—that's how much I love them! (Note: Hachiya persimmons must be fully ripe—the interior should be completely soft and squishy—before they can be eaten; otherwise they're unpleasantly astringent.)

Crust:
1 recipe Cheezcake Crust (p. 212)

Cake:
2 cups (500 mL) cashews
10–11 dates, pitted
5–6 tbsp coconut oil
⅛ tsp salt

½ tsp vanilla
2½ cups (625 mL) chopped Hachiya
  persimmon (nice 'n' ripe!)

1. Soak cashews for 2–4 hours in water and rinse well before using.

2. In a food processor with an s-blade, process dates, oil, and salt to a toffee-like consistency.

3. Add cashews and vanilla and process until smooth.

4. Add persimmons and process until combined well.

5. Pour into pie crust and spread evenly.

Topping:
1½ cups (375 mL) chopped Hachiya
  persimmons (nice 'n' ripe—see note at top)

1. In a blender, purée persimmons, then spread evenly over cake.

2. Chill to set (3–4 hours or overnight).

Makes 1 (10-in [25-cm]) cake.

Desserts

Carrot Cake

Carrot cake—and no flour?! This one was inspired by a star-shaped cake my friend Izumi made for a beach picnic once.

Crust:
½ cup (125 mL) raisins
1½ cups (375 mL) cashews

1. In a bowl, cover raisins with water and soak for ½–2 hours. Reserve ½ cup (125 mL) soaking water for frosting.

2. In a food processor with an s-blade, process cashews to an almost powder consistency, but still crumbly. Set aside in a bowl.

3. In a food processor with an s-blade, purée raisins. Add to bowl and mix thoroughly.

4. Press evenly into bottom of a 10-in (25-cm) springform pan. Set aside.

Cake:
1 cup (250 mL) raisins
15 dates, pitted
¼ cup (60 mL) coconut oil
⅛ tsp ground nutmeg

1½ tsp ground cinnamon
⅛ tsp ground star anise
⅛ tsp ground cloves
10–12 carrots

1. In a bowl, cover and soak raisins for ½–2 hours.

2. In a food processor with an s-blade, purée dates, oil, and ground spices. Set aside in a bowl.

3. In a food processor with a shredding disc, shred carrots. Add to bowl.

4. Add raisins and mix by hand until combined well.

5. Press into pie crust and chill (2 hours) to set.

6. Carefully remove from springform pan and slide onto a large plate to frost.

Frosting:

2 cups (500 mL) cashews

9 dates, pitted

⅛ tsp ground nutmeg

¼ tsp ground cinnamon

⅛ tsp ground cloves

½ cup (125 mL) raisin soaking water

raisins, to garnish (optional)

star anise pods, to garnish (optional)

1. Soak cashews for ½–4 hours and rinse well.

2. In a food processor with an s-blade, process cashews, dates, spices, and water until very smooth and creamy. Set aside in a bowl.

3. With a frosting knife, spread cashew mixture smoothly and evenly over entire cake.

4. Garnish with raisins and star anise pods.

Makes 1 (10-in [25-cm]) cake.

Chocolate Mango Pudding

This creamy whip serves as a pudding, a parfait layer, or a fruit cobbler filling.

2 dates, pitted
1 tbsp coconut oil
¼ cup (60 mL) cacao butter

2 bananas
3 cups (750 mL) chopped fresh mangos

1. In a blender, process dates, oil, cacao butter, and bananas until oil melts.

2. Add mangos and blend just until smooth.

3. Chill to set (3–4 hours).

Makes 3½ cups (830 mL).

Chocolate Strawberry Mango Pudding

This subtly flavored sweet cream serves as a pudding, a parfait layer, or a cobbler filling.

2 dates, pitted
1½ tbsp coconut oil
¼ cup (60 mL) cacao butter
1 banana

1 cup (250 mL) chopped strawberries
2 cups (500 mL) chopped fresh mangos

1. In a blender, process dates, oil, cacao butter, and banana until oil melts.

2. Add strawberries and mangos and blend until smooth.

3. Chill to set (3–4 hours).

Makes 3½ cups (830 mL).

Cobbler Crust

This is a simple base for a cobbler crust that you can use with any number of fillings. The cobbler filling recipes that follow on p. 220 are inspired by my mom's fruit crisps. Cobblers are like a pie, but the fillings don't have to set as stiffly.

1 cup (250 mL) almonds
2 cups (500 mL) sunflower seeds
6–7 dates, pitted

½ tsp salt
2 tbsp coconut oil

1. In a bowl, soak almonds and sunflower seeds for 2 hours or overnight and rinse well before using.

2. In a food processor with an s-blade, process almonds and seeds until sticky but a little chunky. Set aside in bowl.

3. In a food processor with an s-blade, blend dates, salt, and oil until smooth. Add to bowl and mix by hand until well combined.

Makes 4–6 servings.

Fresh Cherry Vanilla Cobbler Filling

You can use any of the many varieties of sweet cherries for this seasonal treat. Serve in a bowl as a cobbler filling or a chunky pudding, or use as a layer in a parfait glass.

5 cups (1¼ L) pitted fresh cherries
1½ bananas
2 dates, pitted
¼ cup (60 mL) coconut oil

½ cup (125 mL) cashews
¼ cup (60 mL) pitted fresh cherries
  (for blending)
⅛ tsp vanilla powder

1. In a food processor with an s-blade, pulse the cherries until diced (or use a knife). Set aside in a bowl.

2. In a blender, process all other ingredients until smooth.

3. Pour over diced cherries and stir to combine well.

Makes 4–5 cups (1–1¼ L).

Mango Coconut Parfait

Alternating with shredded coconut, layer this creamy, fruity mixture into a beautiful glass to create a delicious parfait. It can also be served as a pudding or a cobbler filling.

2 dates, pitted
⅜ cup (90 mL) coconut oil
2 bananas

3¾ cups (935 mL) chopped fresh mangos
½ cup (125 mL) coconut flakes

1. In a blender, process dates, oil, and bananas until oil melts.

2. Add mangos and coconut flakes and blend just until smooth.

3. Chill to set (3–4 hours).

Makes 4 servings.

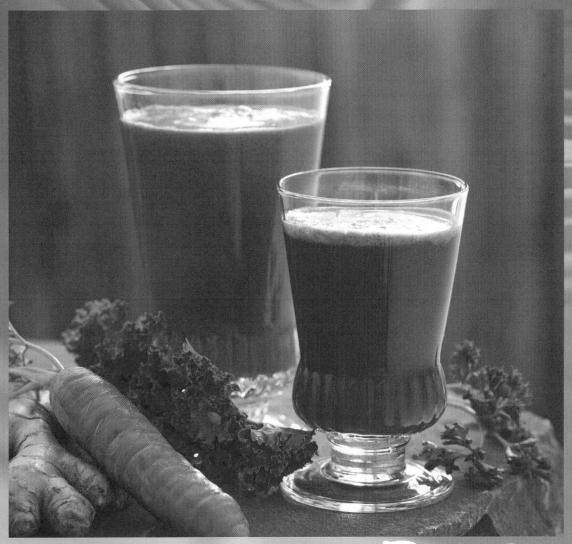

Drinks

Note: I like to use frozen berries and bananas almost always in my blended smoothies and shakes because it makes them cold, thick, and extra creamy without having to use ice. Let your bananas ripen to the perfect sweet spotted stage, then peel them and break them up into 1–2-in (2½–5-cm) pieces before you freeze them.

BC Blue Smoothie

There are several crops that Gorilla Food's home province of British Columbia prides itself on for growing well, and blueberries are one of them.

1–3 tbsp hulled hemp seeds
1–1¼ cups (250–310 mL) orange juice
2 fresh or frozen bananas

½ cup (125 mL) fresh or frozen blueberries

1. In a blender, process all ingredients until smooth.

Makes 1 serving.

BC Blue, Green & Blue Smoothie

A good start to the day! You would hardly know that there is kale in the mix; this is a sweet way to get more greens.

1 tbsp hulled hemp seeds
1–1¼ cups (250–310 mL) orange juice
3–4 kale leaves
2 fresh or frozen bananas

½ cup (125 mL) fresh or frozen blueberries
½ tsp spirulina (optional)

1. In a blender, process all ingredients until smooth.

Makes 1 serving.

Berry Berry Berry Green Smoothie

A fruity smoothie with greens and lots of antioxidants.

⅓ cup (80 mL) fresh or frozen
  blueberries
1⅓ cups (315 mL) fresh or frozen
  strawberries

⅓ cup (80 mL) fresh or frozen
  blackberries
½ tsp açaí berry powder
2 large or 4–5 small kale leaves
1–1¼ cups (250–310 mL) water

1. In a blender, process all ingredients until smooth.

Makes 1 serving.

Helio Tropic Smoothie

Turn to the sun and give thanks!

1 1-in (2½-cm) thick pineapple round
2–3 fresh or frozen bananas
2–4 kale leaves
1–1¼ cups (250–310 mL) orange juice

1. In a blender, process all ingredients until smooth.

Makes 1 serving.

Issa's Electro Lemonade Smoothie

Gorilla Food has a fairy godmother and this is a favorite of hers.

2 lemons, peeled
1½ apples, cored
3 tbsp flax oil
¼ tsp salt
1–1¼ cups (250–310 mL) water

1. In a blender, process all ingredients until smooth.

Makes 1 serving.

Mooney's Goji Zest Smoothie

A re-mixed smoothie from a festival where we had a booth one summer.

½ apple
2 fresh or frozen bananas
½ lemon, peeled
¼ tsp lemon zest
1 tbsp goji berries
1–1¼ cups (250–310 mL) water

1. In a blender, process all ingredients until smooth.

Makes 1 serving.

Simple Green Smoothie

I love how fresh this one is!

1½ apples
2–5 kale leaves
¾ cup (185 mL) chopped fresh or frozen
  strawberries
2 tbsp coconut oil
1–1½ cups (250–310 mL) water

1. In a blender, process all ingredients until smooth.

Makes 1 serving.

Strawberry Electric #9 Smoothie

Filled with energy and, yes, electricity!

1½ fresh or frozen bananas
½ cup (125 mL) chopped fresh or frozen
  strawberries
3 tbsp goji berries
1½ tsp maca powder
1 tsp vanilla powder
½ tsp dried orange zest powder
1–1¼ cups (250–310 mL) water

1. In a blender, process all ingredients until smooth.

Makes 1 serving.

Strawberry Fields Smoothie

One could drink this smoothie forever.

1½ bananas
½ cup (125 mL) chopped fresh or frozen strawberries
1–1¼ cups (250–310 mL) orange juice
1–2 tbsp hemp seeds

1. In a blender, process all ingredients until smooth.

Makes 1 serving.

Strawberry Zing Smoothie

Zip-a-dee-do-da!

1½ bananas
½ cup (125 mL) chopped fresh or frozen strawberries
1–1¼ cups (250–310 mL) orange juice
1 (½–1-in [1–2½-cm]) piece ginger
1–2 tbsp hemp seeds

1. In a blender, process all ingredients until smooth.

Makes 1 serving.

Cherry Berry Electro Lemonade

This was something we served at a great fundraising event with One Yoga for the People and Julia Butterfly Hill benefiting Vinyasa Yoga for Youth. That was fun! What an honor and blessing to serve!

½ cup (125 mL) pitted and chopped fresh
  cherries or dried cherries, soaked
½ cup (125 mL) fresh or frozen
  blueberries
½ date, pitted

1 tbsp goji berries
⅛ tsp salt
⅜ cup (90 mL) lemon juice
1¼ cups (310 mL) water

1. In a blender, purée all ingredients, except water. Pour into a large pitcher, then add water and stir to combine well.

Makes 1 serving.

'Tis the Season Smoothie

One year, during a New Year's break, I mainly drank this green smoothie for a week of cleansing. 'Twas a jolly good season!

4–6 cups (1–1½ L) seasonal greens (kale,
  collards, lettuce, parsley, spinach, etc.)
1½ apples, cored and chopped
2 tbsp flax oil
1 celery stalk, chopped
1–1¼ cups (250–310 mL) water

1. In a blender, process all ingredients until smooth.

Makes 1 serving.

Green Glory Juice

Sweet, green liquid for enlightenment.

1½–2 apples, cored and chopped
½ small–⅓ large lemon, peeled
1 (1-in [2½-cm]) piece ginger
4 celery stalks
¼–⅓ bunch parsley
5 kale leaves
5 seasonal green leaves (collard leaves,
 lettuce leaves, radish tops, etc.)

1. Press all ingredients through a juicer.

Makes 1 serving.

Rawkit Fuel Juice

Enjoy this juice and you'll experience lift off!

2–3 apples, cored and chopped
8 carrots
1 (½–1-in [1–2½-cm]) piece ginger

1. Press all ingredients through a juicer.

Makes 1 serving.

Roots Tonic Juice

Roots give us a connection to the Earth!

⅓–½ medium beet
1 (1-in [2½-cm]) piece ginger
1 4–6-in (10–15-cm) burdock root
8 carrots
¼ cup (60 mL) sunchoke (a.k.a. Jerusalem artichoke)

1. Press all ingredients through a juicer.

Makes 1 serving.

Seasonal Green Juice

Drinking green juice is one of the best things you can do for your body. It may take some getting used to; the first time my friend Lesley served me a straight green juice, it took me all afternoon to get through it. Now I sometimes drink quarts at a time and love it.

1 (1-in [2 1/2-cm]) piece ginger
4–5 celery stalks
½ lemon, peeled
1 cup (250 mL) chopped parsley
4–5 kale leaves

8–10 seasonal green leaves (kale, chard, dandelion, collards, cilantro, etc.)
⅓–½ cucumber

1. Press all ingredients through a juicer.

Makes 1 serving.

Sweet Magenta Juice

Smooth like sylk. May cause instant wake-up and heightened senses!

2 apples
5 carrots
⅓–½ medium beet
1 (½-in [1-cm]) piece ginger (optional)

1. Press all ingredients through a juicer.

Makes 1 serving.

Tropical Twist Juice

The juice formerly known as the Citrus Slinger.

1 (1-in [2½-cm]) thick pineapple round
¾ cup (185 mL) orange juice
1 1-in (2½-cm) piece ginger
3–4 carrots

1. Press all ingredients through a juicer.

Makes 1 serving.

Caro-banan-ananda Shake

I also call this the Hippie Shake.

2–3 fresh or frozen bananas
3 tbsp carob powder
¼ cup (60 mL) almonds
  (dry or sprouted)

1. Press all ingredients through a juicer.

Makes 1 serving.

Note: I like to use frozen bananas almost always in my blended smoothies and shakes because it makes them cold, thick, and extra creamy without having to use ice. Let your bananas ripen to the perfect sweet spotted stage, then peel them and break them up into 1–2-in (2½–5-cm) pieces before you freeze them.

Blackberry Blaze Shake

We have a lot of blackberries in the Vancouver area. They're so good to load up on in summer, and we freeze them for use during winter. Make this a Blueberry Blaze by using blueberries instead.

2–3 fresh or frozen bananas
¼ cup (60 mL) almonds
  (dry or sprouted)
1 date, pitted
1–3 tbsp hemp seeds

1 tbsp coconut oil
1¼ cups (310 mL) water
¾–1 cup (185–250 mL) fresh or frozen
  blackberries (or blueberries)

1. In a blender, process all ingredients until smooth.

Makes 1 serving.

Oh My! Choco Chia Shake

I've tried but I just can't seem to put this shake down until it's finished.

2 tbsp chia seeds
2 tbsp cacao powder
⅛ tsp vanilla powder
2 tbsp cashews

1¼ cups (310 mL) water
3 dates, pitted
1–1½ fresh or frozen bananas

1. In a blender, process all ingredients until smooth.

Makes 1 serving.

Choco Berry Gorilla Shake

The hint of berries adds some fresh fruitiness to this chocolate shake.

2–3 bananas
½ cup (125 mL) fresh or frozen
   blueberries, strawberries, or any
   other berries
¼ cup (60 mL) cacao nibs

¼ cup (60 mL) almonds
   (dry or sprouted)
1 date, pitted
1–3 tbsp hemp seeds
1 tbsp coconut oil
1⅛ cups (280 mL) water

1. In a blender, process all ingredients until smooth.

Makes 1 serving.

Choco Gorilla Shake

Everyday at Gorilla Food, this shake causes people to have the best day ever, over and over!

2–3 fresh or frozen bananas
¼ cup (60 mL) cacao nibs
¼ cup (60 mL) almonds
   (dry or sprouted)

1 date, pitted
1–3 tbsp hemp seeds
1 tbsp coconut oil
1¼ cups (310 mL) water

1. In a blender, process all ingredients until smooth.

Makes 1 serving.

Hempnotic Shake

Hemp can help save the world. It's one of the most underused natural resources on the planet.

2–3 fresh or frozen bananas
1⅛ cups (280 mL) water
¾ cup (185 mL) hemp protein powder

¼ cup (60 mL) almonds
  (dry or sprouted)
1 date, pitted
2–3 tbsp hemp seeds

1. In a blender, process all ingredients until smooth.

Makes 1 serving.

Hempstar Delight Shake

When I was growing up, there was always eggnog during the holiday season. This recipe reminds me of that warm festive feeling.

2–3 fresh or frozen bananas
1⅛ cups (280 mL) water
1–2 tbsp hemp protein powder
¼ cup (60 mL) almonds
  (dry or sprouted)

1 date, pitted
2–3 tbsp hemp seeds
1 (½–1-in [1–2½-cm]) piece ginger
⅛ tsp ground nutmeg
¼ tsp ground cinnamon

1. In a blender, process all ingredients until smooth.

Makes 1 serving.

Strawberry Bliss Up! Shake

A blissing! My favorite shake on the Gorilla Food menu—it's like ice cream.

¼ cup (60 mL) almonds
  (dry or sprouted)
1 date, pitted
1–3 tbsp hemp seeds
1½ fresh or frozen bananas
½ cup (125 mL) chopped fresh or
  frozen strawberries

1¼ cups (310 mL) water
½–1 tsp vanilla powder
1 tbsp coconut oil
1–2 tsp maca powder
¼–½ tsp spirulina

1. In a blender, process all ingredients until smooth.

Makes 1 serving.

Strawberry Cloud Shake

Creamy, sweet, and substantial! The better the strawberries, the better the shake. I love to pour this or the Strawberry Bliss Up! (above) over my grawnola.

¼ cup (60 mL) almonds
  (dry or sprouted)
1 date, pitted
1–3 tbsp hemp seeds

1½ fresh or frozen bananas
½ cup (125 mL) fresh or frozen
  strawberries
1¼ cups (310 mL) water

1. In a blender, process all ingredients until smooth.

Makes 1 serving.

Leo's Lalaland Cardamom & Carrot Sylk

Sunset Boulevard breakfast with L.G. This sylky drink has sweet synchronicity.

1 cup (250 mL) carrot juice
½ cup (125 mL) water
¼ cup (60 mL) almonds
  (dry or sprouted)
2–3 cardamom pods

1. In a blender, process all ingredients until smooth.

Makes 1 serving.

Cashew au Naturel Sylk

Try this unsweetened mylk over grawnola.

¼ cup (60 mL) cashews
1½ cups (375 mL) water

1. In a blender, process all ingredients until smooth.

Makes 1 serving.

Cashew Chocolate Sylk

Add more or less cashews to make it thinner or thicker.

¼ cup (60 mL) cashews   2 dates, pitted
1½ cups (375 mL) water   2 tbsp cacao powder

1. In a blender, process all ingredients until smooth.

Makes 1 serving.

Cashew Vanilla Sylk

Cool, it's refreshing; warm, it's like pudding.

¼ cup (60 mL) cashews   1 date, pitted
1½ cups (375 mL) water   ½ tsp vanilla powder

1. In a blender, process all ingredients until smooth.

Makes 1 serving.

Almond Sylk

When you make your own at home, it's fresh and there are no cartons to throw away.

¼ cup (60 mL) almonds (dry or sprouted)
1¾ cup (415 mL) water

1. In a blender, process all ingredients until smooth.

Makes 1 serving.

Almond Chocolate Sylk

A chocolate variation of the Almond Sylk above.

¼ cup (60 mL) almonds
  (dry or sprouted)

1¾ cup (415 mL) water
2 tbsp cacao powder

1. In a blender, process all ingredients until smooth.

Makes 1 serving.

Almond Vanilla Sylk

I like this with warm water on Grawnola with fruit.

¼ cup (60 mL) almonds
  (dry or sprouted)

1¾ cup (415 mL) water
½ tsp vanilla powder

1. In a blender, process all ingredients until smooth.

Makes 1 serving.

Hemp au Naturel Sylk

A simple, frothy blend from one of the mightiest of plant foods. A good base for a creamy soup, dressing, or sauce too.

5 tbsp hemp seeds
1¾ cups (415 mL) water

1. In a blender, process all ingredients until smooth.

Makes 1 serving.

Hemp Chocolate Sylk

Not too long ago, this drink would have been illegal in Canada and the US. It's got super-foods loaded up in your glass!

¼ cup (60 mL) hemp seeds   1¾ cups (415 mL) water
2 tbsp cacao powder   2 dates, pitted

1. In a blender, process all ingredients until smooth.

Makes 1 serving.

Hemp Vanilla Sylk

I love hemp, but I have so much appreciation for vanilla, too. Together at last!

1¾ cups (415 mL) water   1 date, pitted
¼ cup (60 mL) hemp seeds   ¼ tsp vanilla powder

1. In a blender, process all ingredients until smooth.

Makes 1 serving.

Warm Chai

These spices can be soaked in a jar of water in the sun to make a sun-tea brew, or you can infuse them in warm water. Either enjoy this simple spiced digestive tea on its own or use it to replace the water in any of the Vanilla Sylks (pp. 237-39) to make vanilla chai latte.

2½ tbsp whole cardamom pods
3 tbsp fennel seeds
1 tsp whole cloves
2½ tbsp cinnamon bark chips

2 tbsp dried ground ginger
¾ tsp ground nutmeg
¾ tsp ground black pepper
8 cups water

1. Place cardamon, fennel, cloves, and cinnamon bark in a coffee grinder or high-powered blender and process to almost a powder. Stir into a bowl with ginger, nutmeg, and pepper. Empty into a large glass jar and top with water.

2. Set jar in direct sunlight (e.g., on a windowsill or countertop) for 8–24 hours. Store in the refrigerator.

Makes 8 cups (2 L).

Dark & Spicy Hot Chocolate

This, on a chilly day or night, makes everything alright. If it feels good for the spirit, do you think it's worth a little deviation from the real raw?

2 tbsp cacao powder
3 dates, pitted
2 tbsp chia seeds
¼ cup (60 mL) hemp seeds
¼ tsp ground cinnamon

⅛ tsp ground cayenne
1 tbsp coconut oil
½ tsp vanilla powder
1⅝ cups (400 mL) hot water

1. In a blender, process all ingredients until smooth.

Makes 1 serving.

Earth Resonance Tea

This spice blend came together for an event we did with musician and sound artist David Hickey.

½ cup (125 mL) rooibos tea
⅜ cup (90 mL) peppermint leaves
1 tbsp rosehips
2 tbsp dried St. John's Wort
1 tbsp sarsaparilla root
1 tbsp stevia leaf
1 tsp ground nutmeg
1 tsp vanilla powder

1 tsp ground cinnamon
¼ tsp ground ginger
¼ tsp ground cayenne
2 tbsp maca powder
1 tbsp + 2 tsp carob powder
1 tsp astragalus powder
2 tsp dried nettle leaves

1. In a bowl, mix all ingredients together.

2. Use about 1½ tsp of mix per cup of hot water.

Makes 1½ cups (375 mL).

Goodness Grace Hot Cacao!

Try to put this creamy goodness down. I have a hard time. I hope it warms the heart!

1 heaping tbsp cacao powder
1 tbsp cacao butter
1 tsp coconut oil
¼ tsp vanilla powder

2–3 dates, pitted
⅓ cup (80 mL) cashews
1½ cups (375 mL) warm water

1. In a blender, process all ingredients until smooth, creamy, and frothy.

Makes 1 serving.

Hot Xocolat

This mineral-rich drink is inspired by the chocolate culture of Mexico. There is a long history of cacao drinking in Mesoamerica; research and tasting could fill hours of enjoyable investigation!

3 dates, pitted
2½ cups (625 mL) hot water
2 tbsp cacao powder
⅓ cup (80 mL) sesame seeds

⅛ tsp ground cinnamon
pinch ground cayenne
pinch salt
2 tbsp chia seeds

1. In a blender, process all ingredients until smooth, creamy, and frothy.

Makes 1–2 servings.

Index

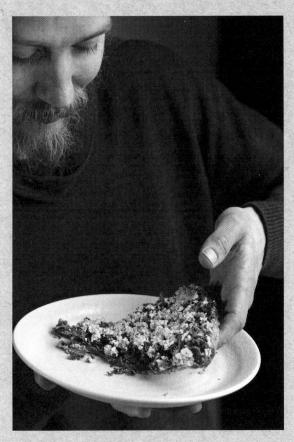

AARON ASH is the founder of Gorilla Food, an organic, vegan, raw food restaurant in downtown Vancouver, Canada that is set to open new locations in fall 2012. He was a personal chef to Mike-D of the Beastie Boys when he lived in Los Angeles. Aaron is also an in-demand caterer for high-profile events around North America.